The Joint Commission

Medication Management made easy

Your Key to Understanding Medication Management in Health Care Settings

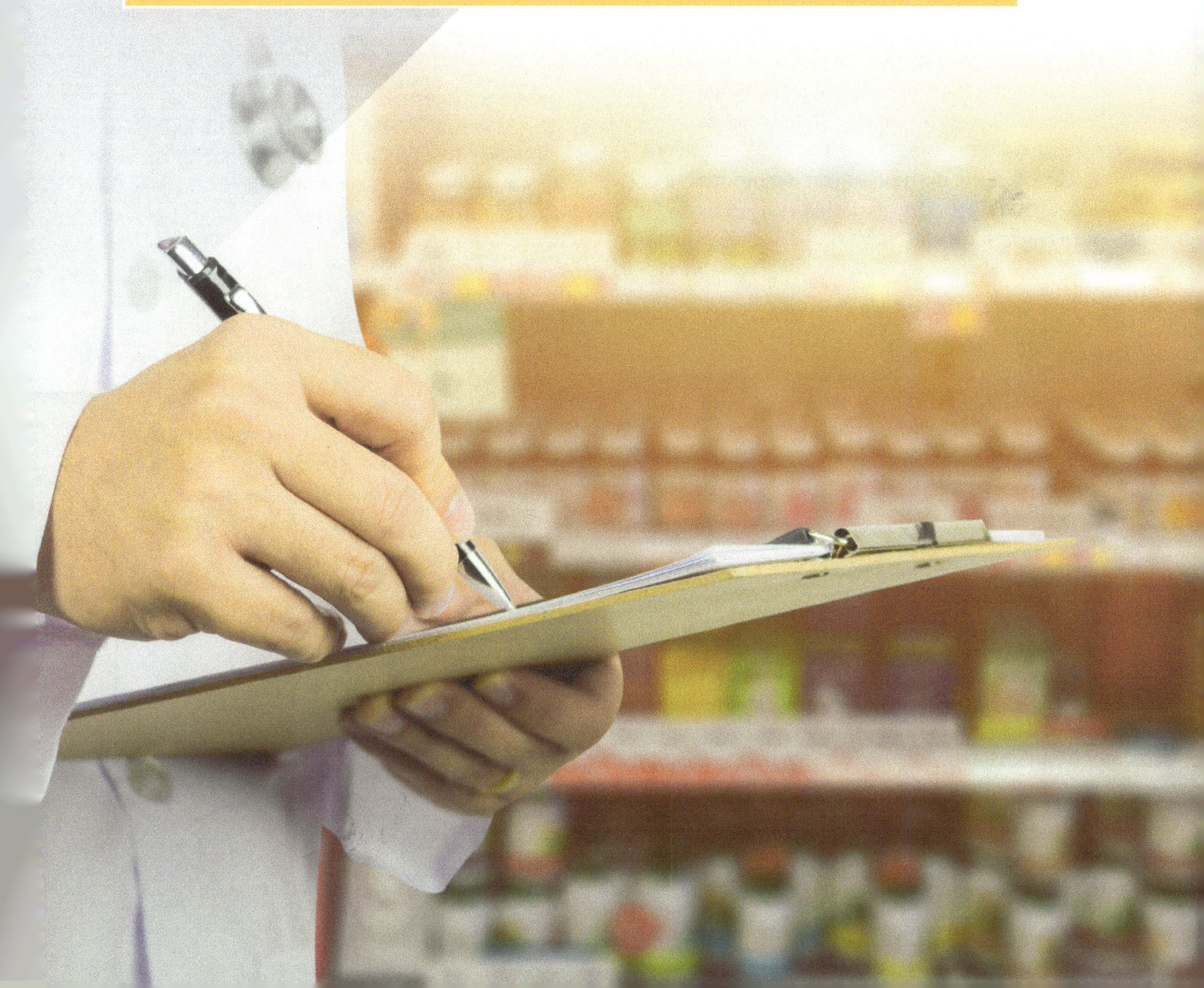

Joint Commission Resources Mission

The mission of Joint Commission Resources (JCR) is to continuously improve the safety and quality of health care in the United States and in the international community through the provision of education, publications, consultation, and evaluation services.

Disclaimers

JCR educational programs and publications support, but are separate from, the accreditation activities of The Joint Commission. Attendees at Joint Commission Resources educational programs and purchasers of JCR publications receive no special consideration or treatment in, or confidential information about, the accreditation process. The inclusion of an organization name, product, or service in a JCR publication should not be construed as an endorsement of such organization, product, or service, nor is failure to include an organization name, product, or service to be construed as disapproval.

This publication is designed to provide accurate and authoritative information regarding the subject matter covered. Every attempt has been made to ensure accuracy at the time of publication; however, please note that laws, regulations, and standards are subject to change. Please also note that some of the examples in this publication are specific to the laws and regulations of the locality of the facility. The information and examples in this publication are provided with the understanding that the publisher is not engaged in providing medical, legal, or other professional advice. If any such assistance is desired, the services of a competent professional person should be sought.

Published by Joint Commission Resources
Oak Brook, Illinois 60523 USA
https://www.jcrinc.com

Joint Commission Resources, Inc. (JCR), a not-for-profit affiliate of The Joint Commission, has been designated by The Joint Commission to publish publications and multimedia products. JCR reproduces and distributes these materials under license from The Joint Commission.

ISBN (print): 978-1-63585-219-6
ISBN (e-book): 978-1-63585-220-2

Printed in the USA

For more information about The Joint Commission, please visit https://www.jointcommission.org.

Development Team

Executive Editor: Mary Beth Curran
Editorial Coordinator: Kristine Stejskal
Associate Director, Global Publications: Helen M. Fry, MA
Associate Director, Production: Johanna Harris
Executive Director, Global Publishing: Catherine Chopp Hinckley, MA, PhD

Reviewers

Joint Commission Division of Accreditation and Certification Operations
Wade Parker, RN, MHA, Field Surveyor
Peter Vance, LPCC, CPHQ, Field Director, Surveyor Management and Development

Joint Commission Division of Business Development, Government, and External Relations
Pearl S. Darling, MBA, Executive Director, Ambulatory Care Services
Julia Finken, BSN, MBA, CPHQ, CSSBB, Executive Director, Behavioral Health Care and Human Services
Gina Zimmermann, Executive Director, Nursing Care Center and Assisted Living Community Services

Joint Commission Division of Healthcare Improvement
Robert Campbell, PharmD, Director, Standards Interpretation Group, and Director, Medication Management

Joint Commission Division of Healthcare Quality Evaluation
Maureen Vance, MSN, RN, Clinical Project Director, Department of Standards and Survey Methods

Joint Commission Resources
Jeannell Mansur, RPh, PharmD, FASHP, FSMSO, CJCP, Principal Consultant, Medication Management and Safety

Office of the General Counsel
Kathleen Pankou, Senior Assistant General Counsel

Table of Contents

Table of Terms

Term	Page	Related Key Concept	Chapter
adverse drug event	28	Written Criteria for Selecting and Procuring Medications	2
adverse drug event	99	Adverse Drug Event Response	7
adverse drug reaction	99	Adverse Drug Event Response	7
antimicrobial resistance	117	Leadership's Commitment to Antimicrobial Stewardship	9
antimicrobial stewardship	117	Leadership's Commitment to Antimicrobial Stewardship	9
automatic dispensing cabinet	74	Dispensing Medications	5
continuum of care	84	Medication Reconciliation	6
controlled medication	41	Medication Control	3
data analysis	107	Analyzing Data	8
emergency medication	38	Safe Storage of Medications	3
family	20	Patient and Staff Engagement and Education	1
floor stock	38	Safe Storage of Medications	3
formulary	28	Written Criteria for Selecting and Procuring Medications	2
hazardous medication	62	High-Alert and Hazardous Medications	4
high-alert medication	62	High-Alert and Hazardous Medications	4
high reliability	23	Common Compliance Challenges	1
high reliability organization	110	Identifying and Addressing Improvement Opportunities	8
infection preventionist	122	Antimicrobial Stewardship Program Elements	9
informed consent	82	Administration Verification Process	6
interdisciplinary	16	Interdisciplinary Approach	1

investigational medication	55	Medication Order Types	4
investigational medication	89	Investigational Medications	6
look-alike/sound-alike medications	58	Look-Alike/Sound-Alike Medications	4
medication control	41	Medication Control	3
medication dose	49	Communicating Medication Orders	4
medication error	99	Adverse Drug Event Response	7
medication frequency	49	Communicating Medication Orders	4
medication management	15	Overview of Medication Management	1
medication outage	32	Medication Shortages and Outages	2
medication reconciliation	84	Medication Reconciliation	6
medication route	49	Communicating Medication Orders	4
medication shortage	32	Medication Shortages and Outages	2
medication substitution	34	Medication Substitution Protocols	2
multidose vial	74	Dispensing Medications	5
PRN medications	49	Communicating Medication Orders	4
protected health information	18	Interdisciplinary Approach	1
psychotropic medication	63	High-Alert and Hazardous Medications	4
qualitative data	107	Collecting Data	8
quantitative data	107	Collecting Data	8
radiopharmaceuticals	41	Medication Control	3
recalled medication	44	Managing Medications in the Inventory	3
risk point	109	Analyzing Data	8
root cause analysis	106	Reporting Requirements	8
self-administration	87	Self-Administration and Medications from Home	6
sentinel event	28	Written Criteria for Selecting and Procuring Medications	2
sentinel event	106	Reporting Requirements	8
side effects	95	Plan to Monitor Patient Response	7
significant adverse drug reaction	99	Adverse Drug Event Response	7
substitution protocol	34	Medication Substitution Protocols	2
therapeutic duplication	67	Reviewing Medication Orders	5
titration orders	56	Medication Order Types	4
tracer methodology	53	Communicating Medication Orders	4

Introduction

Medication management is a complex and interdisciplinary process that involves virtually everyone in a health care organization. An effective medication management system helps organizations ensure that their medications are acquired, stored, ordered, prepared, dispensed, administered, and disposed of in a safe, effective way.

Whether you work at a hospital, nursing care center, home care organization, or other facility, you may be responsible for some facet of the safe and timely delivery of medications. *Medication Management Made Easy* provides an in-depth look at the main components and issues of medication management. We offer tools for implementing a system appropriate to your setting and organization. We also provide a framework for collaboration and education across disciplines and departments, with the goal of continuous improvement.

Each organization is different. Within the framework of laws, regulations, and Joint Commission standards, you need a medication management system—and policies and procedures—that suits your specific setting. For example, a 24-hour inpatient setting needs a dependable medication management system to run without interruption. A home care organization requires a system tailored to the needs of staff members who don't have access to automatic dispensing cabinets. Office-based surgical centers and other outpatient facilities will have their own systems, as will behavioral health care and human services facilities that employ medications that require close monitoring as part of treatment. In other words, not all processes of medication management will apply to every setting or organization.

The health care and human services fields are vast and provide care, treatment, and services to many individuals who may be referred to as patients, individuals served, residents, consumers, or clients. The term patient *is used throughout this book to describe a recipient of care, treatment, and services.*

This Book Focuses on the Basics

We've designed *Medication Management Made Easy* to introduce you to the general principles that underpin an effective medication management system. You'll see how Joint Commission standards provide the foundation for improving—or even designing, planning, and implementing—your own system. This book primarily explores the "Medication Management" (MM) standards of your *Comprehensive Accreditation Manual* or E-dition® counterpart, with the aim of making the requirements approachable, understandable, and actionable (see the sidebar on pages 3–4 for relevant standards from other chapters of the manual). Refer to the *Comprehensive Accreditation Manual* for your setting for a full listing of these standards and for additional information.

The MM standards address the activities and responsibilities of staff and other practitioners across various disciplines within the organization. We provide a big-picture view of the whole system to help you understand how the parts work together. After the individuals involved in planning the medication management system understand how it should function, they can focus on the following key aspects to ensure that the system serves patients safely and effectively:

- Reducing medication variation, errors, and misuse
- Using evidence-based practices to develop effective medication management processes
- Managing processes to promote safe medication management throughout the organization
- Standardizing medication equipment and handling processes across the organization
- Monitoring processes to ensure and improve efficiency, quality, and safety related to medication

This Book Is for You

We developed *Medication Management Made Easy* for five key audiences who either direct, participate in, or support the medication management system within health care organizations: pharmacists or pharmacy technicians, nurses, physicians, or licensed independent practitioners, accreditation professionals, and staff educators.

Although many clinicians don't need to be introduced to the basics of medication management, this book is also a helpful refresher and a resource for clinicians to share with others in their

Relationship to Other Standards

Although *Medication Management Made Easy* focuses primarily on the MM standards, you'll notice cross-references to standards in other chapters in the *Comprehensive Accreditation Manual* or E-dition. The standards are all related. It happens frequently with MM standards. Here's why:

- MM and Record of Care, Treatment, and Services (RC). Medication information must be recorded and updated in the record of care, which is covered by the RC standards.
- MM and Infection Prevention and Control (IC). Safe handling and compounding of medications are part of both medication management and infection prevention and control practice.
- MM and Information Management (IM). Many medical records are stored electronically, which makes them subject to IM standards. A list of prohibited abbreviations for medication documentation and orders is also in the IM chapter (*see* sidebar on page 51). Maintaining the integrity of the record of care and maintaining and adhering to the prohibited abbreviations list are two ways information management contributes to safe medication management.
- MM and Environment of Care (EC). Hazardous medications are disposed of under requirements for disposing of other hazardous materials, as addressed by the EC standards. Recall of medications by federal agencies is also part of the EC team duties.
- MM and Provision of Care, Treatment, and Services (PC) or Care, Treatment, and Services (CTS). Emergency medications, as well as new and self-administered medications, require a heightened focus on the patient's needs, risks, and education and are the domain of the PC and CTS chapters.
- MM and Rights and Responsibilities of the Individual (RI). Pain management and investigational medications, which need to comply with standards related to the rights of the individual, are covered in the RI chapter.
- MM and National Patient Safety Goals (NPSG). These goals cover many patient safety issues, including those related to safe use of anticoagulants, medication reconciliation, and labeling on and off the sterile field in the operating room and procedure areas.
- MM and Leadership (LD). Leadership is responsible for creating a culture that prioritizes safety and is conducive to an environment that is supportive of medication error reporting. LD standards also cover contracted services,

Relationship to Other Standards (continued)

which may be used for pharmacy or other medication-related services.

- MM and Human Resources (HR) or Human Resources Management (HRM). Requirements in these chapters cover many staff competency issues as well as education and training. Staff must have specific skills and knowledge to provide competent medication-related care.

organization who might need a better understanding of the medication management system.

1. **Pharmacists or pharmacy technicians**
   Almost by definition, the pharmacy is the center of medication management activities. You are responsible for acquiring and dispensing medications and, in some cases, for compounding medications. You are responsible for the safe and appropriate provision of medication therapy. You maintain the systems for safe handling and storage of medications, verifying orders, and managing look-alike/sound-alike and high-alert and hazardous medications.

2. **Nurses**
   With rare exceptions, you and other clinical staff members are the ones administering the medication ordered by prescribers and dispensed by pharmacists. You are responsible for the safe and timely administration of those medications to the correct patients. You also monitor patients to ensure the efficacy of medications and to watch for any signs of adverse drug effects.

3. **Physicians or licensed independent practitioners**
   As the primary manager of patients, you need to know which medications are available through your organization's pharmacy or pharmacy partners. You should understand the protocols for ordering and verification, as well as safe handling and administration practices. You also need to understand the medication ordering system employed by your organization to communicate orders to pharmacies. You must know and

adhere to processes related to safety and best practices for handling, administering, and disposing of medications.

4. **Accreditation professionals**
   For the person or part of the team responsible for maintaining your organization's compliance with Joint Commission standards, this book is your entry point to understanding the components of a comprehensive and effective medication management system. Whether your organization is building a system from the ground up or planning to improve an existing system, you can find useful information and tools here to help you ensure that your system is compliant with Joint Commission requirements.

5. **Staff educators**
   As a professional tasked with educating staff about the organization's systems, policies, procedures, and operations, you need a solid understanding of the critical systems in your organization. Medication management is a system that is central to the safe and effective pursuit of the organization's mission. This book offers a foundation of knowledge about the nuts and bolts of medication management processes. It can help you connect the dots to your organization's own medication management system and provide critical information to staff and others who will carry out the processes in their daily work.

This Book Is for All Settings

The medication management system implemented by your organization will vary according to its specific needs and requirements related to the setting of care, including the patient population served, the surrounding community, and other factors. For example, the system needed for medication management at a dialysis center differs substantially from an inpatient psychiatric hospital or a home care provider. These differences are reflected in Joint Commission MM standards for the various settings. Throughout *Medication Management Made Easy*, we note substantial differences in the standards between settings, and we provide tools that have content broad enough to be applicable across settings.

Please note: The Joint Commission Laboratory Accreditation Program does not include MM requirements. Any mention in this book of standards being applicable to certain accreditation programs does not include laboratory settings.

Book Organization and Format

We organized *Medication Management Made Easy* to make it easy for you to find the information and tools you need. We have clearly and consistently labeled and formatted content, and we've identified core content and extra features for targeted reading.

The book is divided into nine chapters that cover major topics addressed by Joint Commission MM standards:

Chapter 1: The Medication Management Program
Chapter 2: Selecting and Procuring Medications
Chapter 3: Safely and Securely Storing Medications
Chapter 4: Ordering and Transcribing Medications
Chapter 5: Preparing and Dispensing Medications
Chapter 6: Administering Medications
Chapter 7: Monitoring Patients' Reactions
Chapter 8: Evaluating the Medication Management Process
Chapter 9: Establishing an Antimicrobial Stewardship Program

Each chapter is organized around several Key Concepts to guide your thinking about these areas of performance. You can access the content as it applies to your organization or as you need it. *Medication Management Made Easy* also includes an appendix of the Medication Management standards and elements of performance (EPs) featured in the book. Please note that these standards and EPs are in effect at the time of publication of this book. Please check your manual or E-dition® for the most up-to-date version.

Chapter features. Within each chapter you will also find recurring features that should help you organize and understand information and relate it to your specific settings and circumstances. These features are listed and explained in this chart.

Chapter Feature	Purpose of Feature
Key Concepts	Highlights key ideas
The Standards	Lists the relevant Joint Commission standards addressed in the chapter and to which programs they apply
In Other Words	Defines key terms in plain language

Chapter Feature	Purpose of Feature
Collaboration	Explains how pharmacists or pharmacy technicians, nurses, physicians or licensed independent practitioners, accreditation professionals, and others can work together
Smart Questions	Provides questions to begin focused conversations on medication management subjects
Picture This	Highlights topics visually
Try This Tool	Lists downloadable, customizable tools and how they can be used
Additional Resources	Offers other resources for the topics discussed in the chapter

In the e-book version of *Medication Management Made Easy*, internal links allow you to easily search for terms and navigate across chapters. Links even take you directly to the downloadable, customizable tools. In the print version, these tools are available online at https://store-jcrinc.ae-admin.com/assets/1/7/MMME21_Landing_Page.pdf.

One note about the tools included in this book: These tools are offered as starting points for thinking about concepts in medication management. You may customize them according to your needs. In recent years, more and more organizations have adopted electronic health records systems, digital pharmacy information and ordering systems, and other information technologies that can perform some of the functions served by these checklists automatically. The tools are included here to help organizations that have not made this transition think about the basics of medication management principles and procedures, but they can also be of use to organizations that have. You may find them useful in evaluating how well your digital solutions are serving your patients and users and where they could be improved to better align with medication management goals.

Acknowledgments

Joint Commission Resources gratefully acknowledges the time and insights of the subject matter experts at The Joint Commission and Joint Commission Resources, who are listed on page ii. We would also like to thank our writer, James K. Foster.

CHAPTER 1

The Medication Management Program

A well-designed medication management program is critical to ensuring that your organization is delivering the right medications, in the right amounts, to the right people in a way that's timely and safe for everyone. The first step to achieving this is to assemble an interdisciplinary team within your organization to break down medication management into smaller processes. The team can then analyze each process—from planning and procurement to staff engagement to patient education and all the steps in between—to identify any points of confusion and areas of potential risk.

Next you'll need to develop policies and procedures to minimize variations and mitigate risk within key processes. Providing clear direction lessens the chances of adverse drug events, medication errors, medication shortages, and other issues and helps make your overall medication management process safer and more reliable.

KEY CONCEPTS

- Overview of Medication Management
- Interdisciplinary Approach
- Patient and Staff Engagement and Education
- Common Compliance Challenges

The Standards

Following are the relevant standards for the content in this chapter from your setting's *Comprehensive Accreditation Manual* or its E-dition® counterpart.

Standard	AHC	ALC	BHC	CAH	HAP	NCC	OBS	OME
IM.02.01.01 The [organization] protects the privacy of health information.	X	X	X	X	X	X	X	X
MM.01.01.01 The [organization] plans its medication management processes.	X	X	X	X	X	X	X	X
MM.05.01.01 [A pharmacist] reviews the appropriateness of all medication orders for medications to be dispensed in the [organization].	X		X	X	X	X	X	X

AHC, Ambulatory Health Care; ALC, Assisted Living Community; BHC, Behavioral Health Care and Human Services; CAH, Critical Access Hospital; HAP, Hospital; IM, Information Managment; MM, Medication Management; NCC, Nursing Care Center; OBS, Office-Based Surgery Practice; OME, Home Care.

The health care and human services fields are vast and provide care, treatment, and services to many individuals who may be referred to as patients, individuals served, residents, consumers, or clients. The term patient *is used throughout this book to describe a recipient of care, treatment, and services.*

KEY CONCEPT

Overview of Medication Management

Anyone who works in health care knows that each patient is unique. And each patient's unique course of treatment is an interdisciplinary process that involves a combination of individuals, from physicians and licensed independent practitioners to nursing staff and pharmacists, just to name a few. With so many people involved in the process, good planning and clear communication are essential to medication safety.

A complete medication management program covers all of your organization's medication processes, which may include the following steps, depending on the care, treatment, and services your organization provides, as well as its size, its patient population, and other factors:

1. Planning
2. Selection and Procurement
3. Storage
4. Ordering
5. Preparing and Dispensing

6. Administration
7. Monitoring
8. Evaluation

We'll dive deeper into each of these processes as we move through this book, but for now here are some basics on what's involved for each area.

picture this

Figure 1-1. Medication Management Process Steps

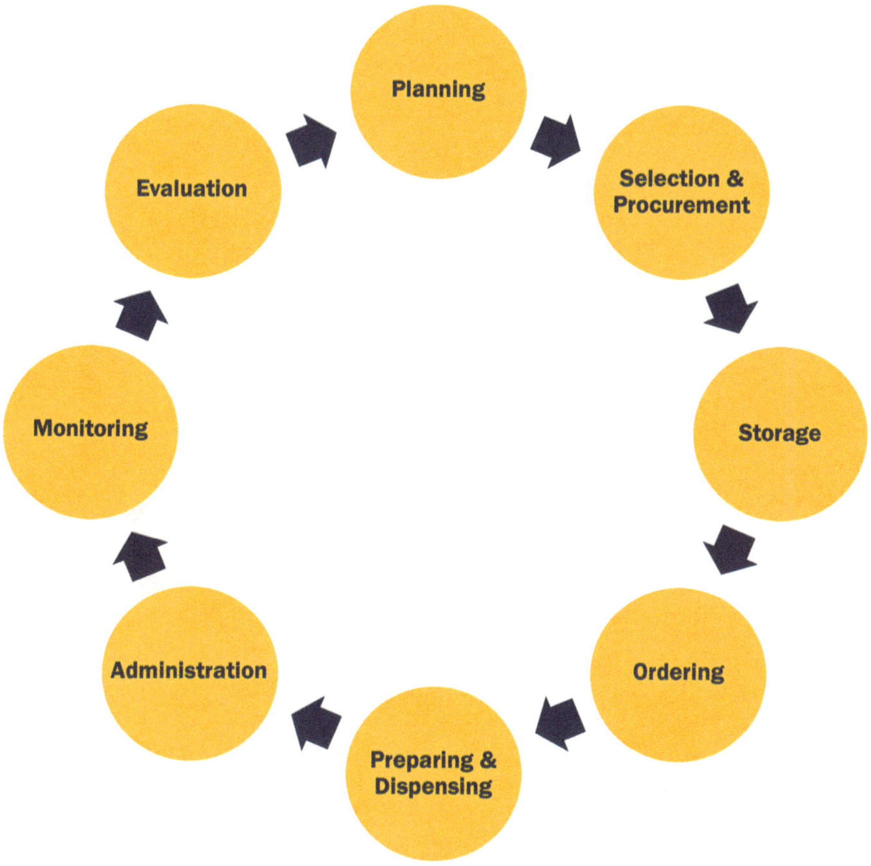

A comprehensive medication management system addresses all of the medication processes of an organization.

Planning

Because every organization and facility is different, there is no one-size-fits-all solution to medication management. As noted above, factors such as size, location, patient population, and the care, treatment, and services offered will affect all aspects of medication management. Some of the questions that may arise during planning include the following:

- Will your organization operate its own 24-hour pharmacy, or will it contract for pharmacy services?
- How will you label or provide special security measures for the medications stored on site?
- Does the organization serve a significant number of individuals who may be self-administering medications?

Asking these and many other questions is just the beginning of your medication management planning activities. You'll want to take each medication process in turn, break it down into its smallest steps, and understand what you need to plan for to make each component function properly.

Collaboration

Any planning activity is an opportunity for collaboration. When assembling an interdisciplinary team to help develop or refine your medication management processes, include representatives from organization leadership, physicians and licensed independent practitioners, nursing staff, pharmacists, the information technology department, and if possible the various specialized departments of your organization (emergency, intensive care, inpatient unit, outpatient services, and so on). This is an opportunity to gain as many perspectives as possible as you gather and share information. It will also help build relationships that will come in handy in the future as you collaborate in other areas of medication management and beyond.

Selection and Procurement

The selection and procurement of medications primarily depends on the types of care, treatment, and services your organization provides and the patient population it serves. You should establish a selection process that takes into account efficacy and side effect research, cost, and availability, as well as administration, storage, safety, and security concerns. Then you need to work with suppliers to ensure a reliable supply of your organization's selected medications, including shipping, handling, emergency planning, possible substitutions, and any other issues that could affect your organization's ability to keep necessary medications in stock.

Storage

Properly storing and keeping track of all the medications in your formulary is no small task. You'll need to make sure that all medications are stored safely and securely, in accordance with law, regulation, manufacturers' instructions, and organization policy. And you'll need to ensure that the medications are available in a timely fashion and in the forms and doses required by those ordering them. This involves not only pharmacy refrigerators but also floor stock areas, automatic dispensing cabinets, emergency carts, and supplies of sample medications. If the medication is for self-administration in the home, you'll need to ensure proper storage there as well.

Ordering

The importance of correctly communicating medication orders cannot be overstated. You need to set up a system that explains who can communicate orders to the pharmacy and what information should be included. Some of the questions to ask include the following:

- What kinds of orders will be allowed?
- What is your preferred method for medication prescribing or ordering?
- Are verbal orders okay?

These and other questions should be addressed during planning. You also should establish procedures for resolving such issues as incomplete or illegible orders so that orders are filled correctly and without delay.

Preparing and Dispensing

Each order that comes into the pharmacy needs to be filled by a qualified staff member. Because proper preparing and dispensing of medications are so central to medication safety, you should give special focus to these areas during planning. A medication management program should cover the facilities and conditions

Smart Questions

What are the most commonly prescribed medications among our patient population?

What less commonly prescribed medications should we carry, and who is in the best position to know this?

What is our process when a medication is ordered or prescribed that is not on our formulary?

What suppliers and vendors are available to provide medications to the organization?

In the event of an emergency, who can supply the organization with essential medications if our primary vendor(s) is unable to do so?

in which medications are prepared in your organization, the elements of proper labeling, a process for reviewing orders, and a process for ensuring that staff members are trained and qualified to perform the functions required of them. These and other aspects of your medication management program may be governed by a variety of rules, laws, and policies.

Although Joint Commission standards are intentionally written to allow organizations a high degree of flexibility in how they design medication management and other systems, more specific guidance and requirements may apply. The Joint Commission recommends referring to the following hierarchy of resources to help guide the design of all aspects of the medication management system:

- Rules and regulations, including state and federal law and regulation
- Conditions of Participation (CoPs) and Conditions for Coverage (CfCs) issued by the Centers for Medicare & Medicaid Services (CMS)
- Manufacturers' instructions for use
- Evidence-based guidelines and national standards
- Consensus documents
- Organization policies

Administration

Medication administration involves getting the correct dose of the correct medication into the correct patient at the correct time and through the correct route. Any policies and procedures that govern this process vary widely by health care setting. For example, home care workers have a different process than staff at a hospital or an opioid treatment clinic. However, no matter the setting, you need to plan how to positively identify patients and correctly match them to their appropriate medications. You also need a program to ensure that staff members who are responsible for administering medications know how to do so properly and understand what to do if they run into any problems or have questions.

Monitoring

Because medication management is central to patient safety and a critical function of many health care organizations, your medication management program should be integrated into any organizationwide performance improvement efforts. Establishing a reporting system that allows staff to provide data on performance, errors, adverse events, near misses, and other variations—as well as the effectiveness of the system as a whole—allows the organization to make candid assessments about what is going well and what is not. How the reporting is done, in what medium, how often, and by whom will vary from organization to organization, but you should have a clear idea of how such monitoring is carried out to make informed decisions toward improving the medication management process.

Evaluation

The final steps involve evaluating your organization's performance information related to medication management, analyzing the data, and presenting the data in ways that provide useful information and insight for leaders. As with any other performance improvement activity, this process should be continuous. The regular search for ways to do better is the

The United States Pharmacopeia

The United States Pharmacopeia (USP) is an independent scientific nonprofit organization that works to ensure the safety, efficacy, and availability of pharmaceutical products. Among its other activities, USP issues standards that cover the safe manufacture, handling, and use of pharmaceuticals. These standards cover a wide variety of related topics, including the safe handling of radiopharmaceuticals and other hazardous substances, sterile compounding of medications at pharmacies, and other areas that touch on aspects of the medication management process.

The Joint Commission is not affiliated with USP, but some of the medication management standards in the *Comprehensive Accreditation Manuals* align with USP standards and will be noted as such with the Joint Commission standard. Remember, compliance with Joint Commission standards is not synonymous with compliance with USP standards. There is some overlap, but you should be familiar with both and understand your responsibilities for each. Also bear in mind that USP is not an enforcement agency. Enforcement of pharmacy regulations is the responsibility of the US Food and Drug Administration (FDA). The Joint Commission ensures compliance with pharmacy regulations during its accreditation process and is a useful resource for medication management best practices.

in other words

medication management

The process an organization uses to provide medication therapy to individuals served by the organization, including procurement, storage, security, prescribing and ordering, transcribing, preparing, dispensing, and administration.

TRY THIS TOOL

Tool 1-1. Medication Management System Stakeholder Analysis Form

This sample form is designed to help you identify component parts of a robust medication management program. Use it to identify relevant organization policies and procedures, compliance issues, the scope of on- and off-site areas of each component, and the individual(s) with the responsibility to address each issue.

hallmark of high reliability organizations. Data analysis, root cause analysis, and other tools can help you find processes that can be improved rather than focusing on individual performance.

KEY CONCEPT

Interdisciplinary Approach

Medication management is inherently an interdisciplinary task. Organization leaders, procurement staff, frontline staff, pharmacists, building engineers, and environment of care specialists are just some of the people who have a role to play in the design of safe and effective medication management.

Leadership

The leaders of an organization are responsible for ensuring that resources are available to procure the appropriate medications and to assist in the enforcement of medication management policies and procedures. Leadership decides how best to apply the available physical, financial, and human resources to the challenges of medication management.

Pharmacy leaders work with staff across the organization to determine the medication needs of the patient populations the organization serves and how best to fulfill those needs. As such, pharmacy leaders are involved in the selection and procurement of medications. What medications will be added to the organization's supply of available medications, and in what quantities? How and from whom will these medications be obtained? In these decisions, pharmacy leaders have to consider the cost of each medication, the needs of the organization's population, possible safety and security issues, and the ease of handling and administration, among other issues.

In addition, pharmacy leaders direct and are intimately involved in monitoring the medication management program. They work with staff, including performance improvement staff, to create ways to monitor and assess how well the process is working. Data from monitoring inform leaders when they are making decisions about how to improve the safety and accuracy of medication management in the organization and how to improve staff training and education.

in other words

interdisciplinary
An approach to care that involves two or more disciplines or professions (for example, social services, specialist consultation, nursing, medicine, therapies, spiritual support) collaborating to plan, treat, or provide care or services to patient and/or that person's family.

Collaboration

As a pharmacist, an accreditation professional, a procurement manager, or anyone else involved in the medication management process, you will likely find that broad interdisciplinary collaboration is important at every step. Medication management is a complex process, and it's important to look at it from as many angles as possible. That said, leadership buy-in—including from medical staff leadership, when applicable—is essential to successful collaboration. After your team considers all of the available information and comes to a decision regarding some aspect of medication management, it's leadership who will make sure that the decision is implemented and its effects monitored.

Procurement Professionals

Procurement professionals specialize in obtaining medications, devices, supplies, and whatever else the organization needs to keep functioning and delivering care, treatment, and services to the people it serves. These professionals are key points of contact with medication suppliers and vendors.

These professionals secure the desired medications, or other goods, in the correct quantities, at the best available prices. They are involved in efforts to reduce waste and inefficiency as supplies are consumed, and they may help provide for the safe and efficient disposal of medication waste products.

Frontline Staff

Physicians, nurses, and other clinicians are central to the medication management program. For example, recommendations from physicians are considered in medication selection decisions, as they come into direct contact with the needs of the patient population. The input of frontline staff in the design and use of the medication ordering system is also essential to ensure the clear and timely communication of orders from prescribers to pharmacists.

Furthermore, because they are responsible for administering medications, frontline staff members are the primary resource for reducing variation in this process to make it safer and more efficient. Finally, these staff members are perhaps best positioned to report on how well the medication management system is serving the patient population.

Simply put, if the medication management program isn't working for frontline staff, it likely is not working at all.

Pharmacy Staff

Pharmacists and pharmacy staff oversee receiving, storing, preparing, and dispensing medications. They are also responsible for reviewing and often managing drug therapy to ensure optimal use of medications. As such, they should be intricately involved in developing the medication management program.

Pharmacists typically are familiar with scientific literature on new therapies and medications, which makes their voices important in selection and procurement decisions. They also can help improve medication ordering and preparation processes. Pharmacists often take the lead in designing the steps for dispensing medications and procedures for such processes as after-hours dispensing and using automatic dispensing cabinets.

In addition, like others involved in the interdisciplinary process, pharmacists and pharmacy staff are great resources for monitoring and performance improvement activities related to medication management.

Engineering Staff

Building engineers, environment of care professionals, and life safety professionals have expertise that contributes to the planning and design of safe work environments for pharmacy staff. They help ensure that the design, layout, and facilities of pharmacy workspaces and medication compounding areas comply with *Life Safety Code*®* and other regulatory requirements and contribute to safe and sterile work practices.

in other **words**

protected health information (PHI)

Health data related to the past, present, or future physical or mental health or condition of an individual; the provision of health care to an individual; or the past, present, or future payment for the provision of health care to an individual.

TRY THIS TOOL

Tool 1-2. Accessibility of Patient Information Policy

This sample policy addresses the need for basic patient information to be accessible to staff involved in medication management processes, as well as steps for safeguarding that information from improper disclosure.

---

* *Life Safety Code*® is a registered trademark of the National Fire Protection Association, Quincy, MA.

KEY CONCEPT

Patient and Staff Engagement and Education

Among the most important aspects of medication management are patient and staff engagement and education. It's easy to get focused during the planning stages on the myriad departments and units of your organization that take part in medication management. However, keep in mind that patients are the ones on the receiving end, and therefore it is essential to involve them in the process as much as possible.

For some organizations, this need will be more obvious. For instance, ambulatory health care, behavioral health care and human services, and home care organizations often deal with patients or clients who self-administer medications. These individuals, and/or their family members, will need thorough education on how to safely store and administer medications and how to monitor for efficacy and adverse reactions.

Patient Engagement

Patient medication engagement is the process of getting patients and/or their caregivers involved in managing their own medications. This can be done in a number of ways. In outpatient settings, patients are responsible for administering their medications, monitoring their conditions, and looking out for and reporting adverse drug reactions. It's important in these settings to maintain regular contact with patients by scheduling regular follow-up appointments, which can be done by phone, e-mail, or text. Maintaining multichannel communication, such as phone calls, e-mails, and mailed correspondence, with patients in outpatient care also helps ensure that patients show up for in-person appointments and follow through on contacts with other providers.

For inpatient environments, one of the best ways to engage patients in medication management is to have regular conversations with them about how well their medications are working, if they are experiencing any side effects (and how severe the effects are), and what alternative medications are available to them. To help support self-administration of medications for patients when they return home, you may want to provide other resources, such as checklists and forms or apps and websites, to help patients track self-administration, medication effects and side effects, usage patterns, adverse reactions, and other useful data. These data can then inform future conversations between patients and their care team about next steps in the plan for care, treatment, or services.

During these conversations it is important to respect cultural and religious differences. Engagement between patients, caregivers, nurses, and practitioners is key to understanding cultural, religious, and other factors that may affect how patients and their families make health care decisions.

Patient Education

Patients and/or their families need clear and timely information to make the best decisions available to them. They need to know why medications are being prescribed, the possible risks and benefits of each medication, and any alternatives to medication that might be available. The Joint Commission's Provision of Care, Treatment, and Services (PC) standards (or Care, Treatment, and Services [CTS] standards in behavioral health care care and human services settings) require that organizations educate patients about the safe and effective use of medications and that they take concrete steps to make sure this information is understood by the patient and/or families. This ensures that patients and their families can make informed decisions about their care, including decisions about which medications the patient should be given. More specifically, PC standards for nursing care centers require organizations to provide education for patients and family members on, among other topics, the risks, benefits, and use of psychotropic medications.

It is critical to convey as much information about medications being taken as possible to patients and/or families using clear language. Patients with limited English proficiency or low levels of health literacy may need additional educational materials or interpretation services. With clear and effective patient education tools, patients and their families can become indispensable sources of information when deciding on the best course of treatment.

in other words

family

A person or persons who play a significant role in an individual's life. A family is a group of two or more persons united by blood or adoptive, marital, domestic partnership, or other legal ties. The family may also be a person or persons not legally related to the individual (such as a significant other, friend, support person, or caregiver) whom the individual personally considers to be family. A family member may be the surrogate decision-maker if authorized to make care decisions for the individual should he or she lose decision-making capacity or choose to delegate decision making to another.

Staff Engagement and Education

Keeping staff members engaged in their job and their role in medication management are key ways to increase reliability and safety across your organization. There are many ways to encourage and support staff engagement, including the following:

- Fostering a culture of safety and accountability, where errors are an opportunity to improve processes rather than lay blame, and staff members feel comfortable suggesting improvements to processes

- Managing workloads through adequate staffing levels and good process design
- Nurturing trust and a team-oriented atmosphere that emphasizes high standards and levels of accountability, as well as mutual support
- Encouraging communication in all phases of the medication management process, including communication with patients, other staff members, pharmacists, and leadership
- Setting clear expectations and providing actionable feedback through assessment
- Supporting a healthy work-life balance that helps prevent employee burnout

TRY THIS TOOL

Tool 1-3. Patient Medication Education Checklist

Use this checklist to plan for what kinds of patient education you will provide, when, and what materials or other support you will provide patients and their caregivers.

In addition to supporting staff engagement, the complexity of the medication management system demands robust staff education. Staff must know their roles as they pertain to all aspects of the medication management program. Initial training and ongoing education should focus on providing staff with a clear idea of what their responsibilities are; the content of the organization's various medication management protocols, policies, and procedures; and their responsibilities under law and regulation. Data gathered through performance monitoring and improvement activities can be an invaluable tool in designing continuing staff education programs that support improvement in specific areas.

KEY CONCEPT

Common Compliance Challenges

A continuous process of monitoring and improvement activities can help organizations on their way toward higher reliability and greater medication safety. During this process you will identify aspects of the medication management system that present greater or more persistent challenges. To help you start thinking about areas for improvement, this section presents some of the medication management standards that are most commonly scored by Joint Commission surveyors, along with approaches to improving compliance with these standards.

Safe Storage of Medications

Medication Management (MM) Standard MM.03.01.01 is among the most commonly scored standards on surveys, across all settings, for the last several years. It is the standard that requires the safe storage of medications.

What's the problem? The challenge is twofold. Many medications need to be stored under specific conditions of temperature, humidity, and other factors to continue to be safe and effective. Home care organizations may find that a patient's home lacks consistent refrigeration or climate control and may need to find another place to store a patient's medications. Hospitals and other facilities storing some vaccines and other medications may find they need to invest in ultracold freezers. They also need a way to verify that proper temperatures are or have been maintained for all medications in locations that may be closed on weekends or holidays.

In addition, procedures for safely storing medications may be complicated and time consuming. This can sometimes lead to staff using shortcuts or workarounds that introduce variation into the process.

Why do I need to know this now? The frequency with which this standard is scored suggests that it is a persistent challenge across health care settings. The fact that improperly stored medications may expire, become contaminated, or lose efficacy represents an increased risk to patient safety.

Where do I start? Start by collecting and organizing information about what steps of this process your organization is doing well and where things could be improved. Some questions to ask to get you started include the following:

- What are all the locations where medications are stored? What are the official medication storage areas in the facility?
- Are all medications stored according to manufacturers' recommendations or the pharmacist's instructions?
- Are controlled substances properly secured according to law and regulation?
- Does our organization have a comprehensive medication control policy that addresses the control of medications from receipt through administration and covers safe storage, handling, security, wasting, disposition, and return to storage?
- What measures are we taking to ensure against access to medications by unauthorized persons?
- Are all medications and their components properly labeled with the contents, expiration date, and any applicable warnings?

- Are all expired, damaged, or contaminated medications removed from the regular storage area and stored separately?
- How often do we inspect medication storage areas, particularly those outside our facilities?

Pharmacist Review of Medication Orders

Another MM standard that is among the most commonly scored on surveys in recent years is MM.05.01.01: [A pharmacist] reviews the appropriateness of all medication orders or prescriptions for medications to be dispensed in the [organization].*

What's the problem? Pharmacies are busy places, and pharmacists are busy people. In addition, not all organizations have a pharmacist on staff or access to a pharmacist 24 hours a day, 7 days a week. Furthermore, an on-call pharmacist may be working with several organizations at once, or a pharmacist may be new to an organization and may not be familiar with the organization's ordering policies. These and other factors can cause staff to skip steps in the process in order to fulfill patients' medication needs quickly or to just lack some of the information they need.

Why do I need to know this now? The pharmacist review requirement is a patient safety measure. It's a critical point in the ordering process, where a qualified individual ensures the accuracy and appropriateness of the order for the individual who will receive the medication.

Where do I start? Start by asking questions about your process. Scoring on this standard tends to focus on two areas: Element of Performance (EP) 4, which sets out the minimum requirements of the pharmacist review, and EP 11, which requires all concerns, issues, or questions to be clarified or resolved with the prescriber before the medication can be dispensed. A few questions to start with include the following:

- Does our organization employ or contract with a pharmacist who can perform this order review whenever it is needed?
- Do staff and prescribers know how to contact a pharmacist during off-hours and when off site?
- Are all reviewing pharmacists aware of the minimum requirements of the review?

in other **words**

high reliability

Consistent excellence in quality and safety across all services maintained over long periods of time.

TRY THIS TOOL

Tool 1-4. Medication Storage and Security Assessment Checklist

We'll dig deeper into safe and secure storage of medications in Chapter 3, but if you are interested in assessing your organization's medication storage security, this checklist is a good place to start.

* There are exceptions related to who conducts this review in different settings. See your setting's *Comprehensive Accreditation Manual* or its E-dition counterpart for specific requirements.

- Does our medication management policy allow for sufficient time to resolve issues with orders?
- What is the organization's policy addressing how pharmacists should contact prescribers when they need clarification or help resolving issues with orders?

Medication management is a complex system made up of interlocking processes that spread across an organization. To succeed, you'll need to assemble an interdisciplinary team to break the program into smaller processes. Then you can analyze each process to see where the risk factors are and decide how to address them. Solid planning and monitoring of the program, including practices that reduce variation and confusion, are keys to success. In-person interaction and training can be critical tools for ensuring that anyone who works with medications, including pharmacy staff, physicians, nurses, and therapists, are aware of organizations' medication ordering policies and other relevant information.

Additional Resources

- US Food and Drug Administration (FDA) ensures that safe and effective medications are available to improve the health of people in the United States. https://www.fda.gov/
- Health Insurance Portability and Accountability Act (HIPAA) addresses the protected health information (PHI) handled and distributed during the medication management process. https://www.hhs.gov/hipaa/for-professionals/privacy/laws-regulations/index.html
- United States Pharmacopeia (USP) is an independent scientific nonprofit organization that works to ensure the safety, efficacy, and availability of pharmaceutical products. https://www.usp.org/

CHAPTER 2

Selecting and Procuring Medications

The medication needs and capabilities of every organization are different. As a first step, your organization needs to decide which medications it will have available based on the patient population it serves and the organization's mission. After this is determined, you need to create—and regularly update—a list of all the medications that are approved for use, as well as plan for shortages or outages by developing medication substitution protocols. Just like many of the processes surrounding medication management, the selection and procurement process is a collaborative effort involving leadership, pharmacists, licensed independent practitioners and physicians, respiratory therapists, and nurses, among other clinical staff.

KEY CONCEPTS

- Written Criteria for Selecting and Procuring Medications
- Creating and Maintaining a Formulary
- Medication Shortages and Outages
- Medication Substitution Protocols

The Standards

Following are the relevant standards for the content in this chapter from your setting's *Comprehensive Accreditation Manual* or its E-dition® counterpart.

Standard	AHC	ALC	BHC	CAH	HAP	NCC	OBS	OME
EM.02.01.01 The [organization] has an [Emergency Operations Plan].	X	X	X	X	X	X	X	X
EM.02.02.03 As part of its [Emergency Operations Plan], the [organization] prepares for how it will manage resources and assets during emergencies.	X	X	X	X	X	X	X	X
MM.02.01.01 The [organization] selects and procures medications.	X		X	X	X		X	X

AHC, Ambulatory Health Care; ALC, Assisted Living Community; BHC, Behavioral Health Care and Human Services; CAH, Critical Access Hospital; EM, Emergency Management; HAP, Hospital; MM, Medication Management; NCC, Nursing Care Center; OBS, Office-Based Surgery Practice; OME, Home Care.

The health care and human services fields are vast and provide care, treatment, and services to many individuals who may be referred to as patients, individuals served, residents, consumers, or clients. The term patient *is used throughout this book to describe a recipient of care, treatment, and services.*

KEY CONCEPT

Written Criteria for Selecting and Procuring Medications

One of the first tasks for your medication management team is the creation of written criteria that govern which medications your organization will make available and the criteria you will use to select them. In hospitals and large health care organizations, this work is generally done by a standing committee, such as a Pharmacy and Therapeutics Committee. This committee may report to the hospital's board, either directly or through another committee. In smaller organizations, an individual or a small group may handle this task.

Joint Commission standards vary somewhat on this topic according to the health care setting. For instance, behavioral health care and human services standards are less specific about who must be involved in creating the written criteria, although the standards are generally consistent across settings when it comes to the minimum requirements. Still, it is a good idea to get as many points of view as possible.

In general, if your organization is a hospital or another entity that operates a pharmacy, the criteria for deciding which medications you will carry must include, at a minimum, the following:

- **Indications for use**
  - What is the medication for?
  - Does the medication address the needs of patients?
  - Does your patient population have a need for this medication?
- **Effectiveness**
  - How well does the medication address the needs of patients?
  - Are there other medications that would work better? If so, what are they?
  - What do practitioners, nurses, and the literature have to say about the effectiveness of specific medications?
- **Drug interactions**
  - What is the potential for adverse reactions between the medication and other medications, particularly commonly prescribed ones, in the organization's formulary?
- **Potential for errors and abuse**
  - Is this medication a high-alert medication (such as insulin) that could be particularly harmful to patients if used in error?
  - Is this medication a controlled substance that would present an elevated risk of abuse?
  - Is this medication a look-alike/sound-alike medication that is likely to be confused with other medications in the organization's formulary?
- **Adverse drug events**
  - What data are provided on likely (common), rare, or serious side effects?
  - How does the side effect profile compare with other medications used to treat the same condition?
- **Sentinel events**
  - Is there a sentinel event regarding this medication? (See sidebar on page 28.)
  - Has the medication been associated with one or more sentinel events in your organization?
- **Population served**
  - Given the population your organization serves, how likely are you to need to prescribe this medication?
  - Does your organization serve special populations (the elderly, children, families, pregnant women and newborns, trauma patients)? (These and other populations may need specific medications or types of medications.)

- **Other risks**
  - Is the medication hazardous?
  - Do you have a mechanism to store the medication or prepare it in a way that is safe and conforms to law, regulation, and manufacturer's instructions?
  - Does the medication require special handling, such as very cold storage?
- **Costs**
  - What are the costs associated with the medication? (This may include information about any associated costs related to special handling or security; special materials or devices for storage, preparation, and administration; and special procedures for disposal of expired medications and related waste.)
  - How does this cost per day/cost per treatment compare with other available medications on the formulary used to treat this condition?

You can see the importance of getting input from across the organization on medication procurement decisions when you review the above points (see Figure 2-1 on page 29). Each of these considerations touches on a slightly different area of the organization's operations and expertise.

in other words

adverse drug event

An injury resulting from a medical intervention related to a medication, including harm from an adverse drug reaction or a medication error. *See also* medication error.

formulary

A written list of all the medications an organization makes available to be prescribed and administered to patients.

sentinel event

A patient safety event (not primarily related to the natural course of the patient's illness or underlying condition) that reaches a patient and results in death, permanent harm, or severe temporary harm. Sentinel events are a subcategory of adverse events.

TRY THIS TOOL

Tool 2-1. Medication Selection Criteria Worksheet

Use this worksheet to help you ask the right questions about and weigh the pros and cons of each medication you are considering having available in your organization.

Medication-Related Sentinel Events

To help organizations increase patient safety, The Joint Commission regularly issues *Sentinel Event Alerts*. These newsletters identify specific kinds of sentinel and adverse events and high-risk conditions and their common root causes. They also suggest evidence-based strategies for reducing the risk of future occurrence.

The following are current *Sentinel Event Alerts* from The Joint Commission that relate to medication management. Visit https://www.jointcommission.org/resources/patient-safety-topics/sentinel-event/ to download PDFs of the literature for these and other *Sentinel Event Alerts*.

- *Sentinel Event Alert* 39: Preventing pediatric medication errors
- *Sentinel Event Alert* 61: Managing the risks of direct oral anticoagulants

picture this

Figure 2-1. Interdisciplinary Team for Medication Selection and Procurement

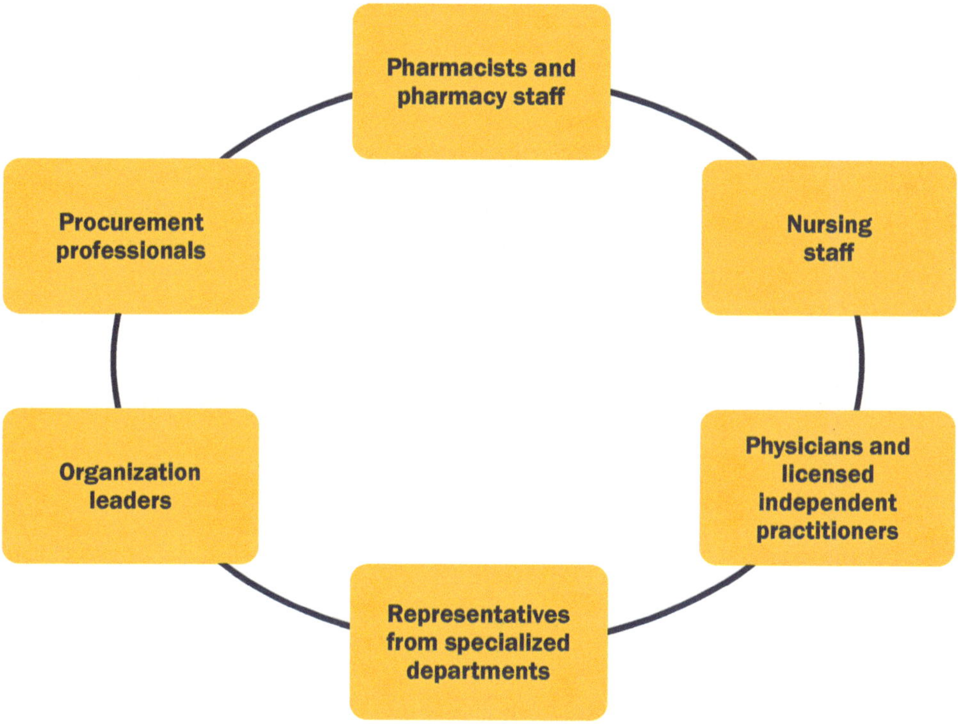

Selecting and procuring medications are important processes that require individuals in different disciplines in the organization to work closely together.

KEY CONCEPT

Creating and Maintaining a Formulary

Joint Commission Medication Management (MM) Standard MM.02.01.01, Element of Performance (EP) 4, requires organizations to maintain a formulary—that is, a written list of all medications the organization makes available to be prescribed and administered. Although this is required only for hospitals, critical access hospitals, ambulatory health care centers, and home care organizations, it is a good idea for any organization that prescribes medications.

The formulary should include the brand names and generic names of each medication, along with the dosage and strength information and the standard concentrations in which each medication is available. Be sure to make this list easily accessible to anyone involved in the medication management process, from procurement through preparation and dispensing to administration and disposal of waste. **Note:** You are not required to include sample medications on the formulary.

Adding and Removing Medications

Don't think your work is done when your organization has developed a formulary. The formulary is not a static document. You need to develop a system for how to make decisions related to selecting, approving, and procuring new medications to add to the formulary and, when necessary, to remove from the list. As noted above, in larger organizations and hospitals, this work is typically done by a standing committee. Smaller organizations need to create a formulary review process that works for them.

Review the formulary at least annually, considering emerging safety and efficacy information about each medication on the list. During the review, make time to discuss new and newly available medications, their safety and efficacy, and their appropriateness for your organization. This review, as well as a review of the formulary decision-making process itself, will help your organization stock the safest and most appropriate medications available, in the best dosages, concentrations, and forms to serve your patient population.

Automating Procurement Functions

As technology evolves and more organizations turn to digital inventory control systems, there is an opportunity to automate procurement functions. Although automation can make the management of any process go more smoothly, it also makes the periodic review of such processes all the more important, as automation can encourage a kind of "set-it-and-forget-it" approach.

Remember, Joint Commission standards don't address medication inventory control systems; rather, organizations can select or design these systems to suit their needs. Depending on the health care setting, MM.02.01.01 does require organizations to maintain a formulary (EP 4) and to follow a process for selecting, approving, and procuring medications that are not on its formulary (EP 7). If you choose to integrate formulary functions and inventory control systems, remember that they are distinct functions for purposes of compliance.

Collaboration

Creating and maintaining a formulary presents another opportunity to bring together your medication management team. Just as you collaborated across your organization to implement a medication management program, it is important to bring stakeholders together again to assess how it is working. Are the goals your team set being achieved? What changes to the system are necessary?

Bring in data specialists, if you have access to them, to help you understand how well your procurement system is meeting the needs of your patients. These specialists can help suggest areas for improvement. Together, you can collectively decide on actions to improve efficiency, effectiveness, and ease of use.

KEY CONCEPT

Medication Shortages and Outages

Health care organizations experience occasional shortages or outages of certain medications. Sometimes, such as during an emergency, the whole medication supply chain may be disrupted. Your organization must develop a process for communicating shortages or outages of specific medications, or of the medication supply chain in general, to prescribers and other staff involved in medication management.

Alerting Prescribers to Shortages and Outages

When deciding how to communicate a medication shortage or outage, first account for the severity and predicted duration of the shortage or outage, as well as its scope. For example, there is no need to alert the entire staff that your organization has depleted its supply of a medication that is commonly used by only a handful of practitioners or administered to a relatively small number of patients.

TRY THIS TOOL

Tool 2-2. Formulary Worksheet

Use this worksheet to record brand and generic names, appropriate dosages and strengths, and any other notes and concerns for each medication on your formulary.

Smart Questions

What is the process for adding or removing medications from the formulary or list of medications available for use?

Who is involved in making decisions about medication selection and procurement?

If your organization does not operate its own pharmacy, where do you turn for pharmacist input on decisions about what medications you will make available to your patients?

Who has the authority to make changes to the formulary?

How is the formulary made available to those who use the medication system? How are changes to the formulary shared after decisions are made?

Those involved in the planning and implementation of changes to the medication management program may work with information management professionals in your organization to devise a system that is responsive and can scale up for shortages and outages that are longer or broader in their impact. Perhaps, for instance, reports could identify the most frequent prescribers of a medication that is in short supply so that updates can be provided directly to those prescribers. As another option, all order sets that include the medication in short supply can be identified so that a substitute medication can be included.

in other words

medication outage
A period of time when the supply of a medication has been completely depleted.

medication shortage
A period of time when the demand or projected demand for a medication exceeds the supply of the medication.

Smart Questions

What are your criteria for declaring a medication shortage or outage?

How do you notify prescribing staff when a shortage or outage occurs or ends?

How do you alert nurses and frontline staff about a shortage or an outage?

How do you proactively monitor for medication shortages or outages to prevent the disruption of care, treatment, or services?

What other strategies do you employ when a shortage or an outage exists (for example, alternative medications, rationing according to criteria developed by pharmacy and medical staff, and so on)?

Where will the organization acquire medications if its primary supplier cannot provide them?

Having a Backup Plan

Whether they are due to a communitywide emergency, a supply chain disruption, or a cause that is narrower in scope, some medication outages may last weeks or more. For shortages caused by external disasters such as hurricanes, you probably already have a plan in place to respond to these situations. All Joint Commission–accredited organizations are required under Emergency Management (EM) Standard EM.02.01.01 to have an Emergency Operations Plan (EOP) or Emergency Management Plan. The EOP contains plans for how to ensure that a supply of medications, including commonly used substitutes if necessary, are available in the case of a medication outage (EM.02.02.03, EP 1). If your organization employs a full-time emergency management professional, consult with him or her for ideas on how to keep the organization properly supplied with medications.

In addition to identifying alternative sources for medications, you should also make sure that you have contingency plans to guarantee the delivery of medications from primary or alternative suppliers to your organization, in case shortages or outages are caused by physical or logistical obstacles such as blocked or closed roads or a shortage of vehicles or personnel or other circumstances that are out of your control.

KEY CONCEPT

Medication Substitution Protocols

When there is a prolonged shortage or outage of a needed medication, it may be possible to substitute another medication of which the organization has a greater supply. Your organization will need to think carefully about when and how to do this and come up with written protocols that cover this process.

Following are some issues your medication substitution protocols should address.

Law and Regulation

Your organization needs to meet state laws and regulations addressing medication substitution allowances. These laws can vary substantially from state to state, as well as by drug class and the type of organization. What may be legal or permissible for hospitals that operate their own pharmacies may not be okay for home care organizations. For example, behavioral health care and human services organizations that provide controlled substances as part of therapy will be subject to different laws and regulations than those that don't.

Possible Drug Interactions

The substitution of one or more medications for another may raise the possibility of new or different drug interactions, which can lead to the risk of an adverse event. Identify in your medication substitution protocols who can make the decision to authorize such substitutions. In hospitals medical staff must approve any outages and substitutions declared by the chief pharmacist, and the declaration typically has to be approved by the Pharmacy and Therapeutics Committee or a similar body.

When an outage or a shortage is declared, the pharmacist consults with physicians to identify a list of acceptable substitutes that includes information about possible adverse interactions and other relevant safety information. Some or all of this information can be integrated into an electronic ordering system to further reduce variation and the probability of error. In any case, extra vigilance is warranted whenever these kinds of substitutions occur.

Staff Roles During a Shortage or an Outage

When a shortage or an outage is declared by pharmacy leadership, your organization's written medication substitution protocols should also identify who receives this information and how. Include in the protocols a process for communicating substitutions due to outages or shortages to licensed independent practitioners and staff involved in your medication management program, along with any required training to frontline staff on different administration requirements and how to monitor effects and side effects.

TRY THIS TOOL

Tool 2-3. Medication Outage or Shortage Substitution Protocols

These sample protocols address how to safely use substitute medications during a medication shortage or outage. Adapt the protocols to suit the needs and requirements of your organization.

in other words

medication substitution
The practice of replacing a prescribed medication with a different medication that is expected to have the same clinical effect.

substitution protocol
The procedures and rules that govern the use of one or more medications instead of another medication, including the roles and responsibilities of pharmacists and other staff to document the substitution and communicate it to appropriate staff. Substitutions may be called for during shortages or outages, but they may also occur for therapeutic reasons or because of cost, as in the case of generic substitutions.

If possible, use information from electronic health records and digital ordering systems to identify prescribers whose orders will be affected by the substitution. Physicians, in turn, will work with pharmacists to identify acceptable available substitute medications, and those decisions will be reflected in ordering software or procedures. How exactly this happens will vary by organization and setting. Standard MM.02.01.01, EP 12, only requires that you have protocols to address it.

The medication selection and procurement system ties directly into your organization's core mission to provide high-quality care, treatment, and services to your patient population. Establishing clear, efficient processes for identifying and obtaining medications, as well as planning for medication shortages and outages, are critical steps toward ensuring that your organization can provide the best available medications to those who need them.

Additional Resources

- The Centers for Medicare & Medicaid Services (CMS) provides a web page for formulary guidance, including information on prescription medication coverage policies under Medicare. https://www.cms.gov/Medicare/Prescription-Drug-Coverage/PrescriptionDrugCovContra/RxContracting_FormularyGuidance
- The US Food and Drug Administration (FDA) provides guidance to commonly asked questions by formulary committees and similar entities about prescription medications and devices. https://www.fda.gov/regulatory-information/search-fda-guidance-documents/drug-and-device-manufacturer-communications-payors-formulary-committees-and-similar-entities

CHAPTER 3

Safely and Securely Storing Medications

Organizations that dispense medications need to prioritize safe and secure storage to help ensure the safety of patients, staff, and visitors. Secure storage, along with robust tracking and controlling access to medications, is a critical part of medication management.

Another key aspect of the safe storage of medications is the removal of expired, damaged, or contaminated medications from circulation and separating such medications from those that are still usable. Furthermore, retrieving and returning recalled medications in accordance with law, regulation, and organization policy enhances patient safety. Strong medication management and oversight are critical to these efforts.

KEY CONCEPTS

- Safe Storage of Medications
- Medication Control
- Managing Medications in the Inventory

The Standards

Following are the relevant standards for the content in this chapter from your setting's *Comprehensive Accreditation Manual* or its E-dition® counterpart.

Standard	AHC	ALC	BHC	CAH	HAP	NCC	OBS	OME
MM.03.01.01 The [organization] safely stores medications.	X	X	X	X	X	X	X	X
MM.03.01.03 The [organization] safely manages emergency medications.	X	X	X	X	X	X	X	X
MM.03.01.05 The [organization] safely controls medications brought into the [organization] by patients, their families, or licensed independent practitioners.	X	X	X	X	X	X	X	X
MM.05.01.11 The [organization] safely dispenses medications.	X		X	X	X		X	X
MM.05.01.17 The [organization] follows a process to retrieve recalled or discontinued medications.	X		X	X	X	X	X	X
MM.05.01.19 The [organization] safely manages returned medications.	X	X	X	X	X	X		X

AHC, Ambulatory Health Care; ALC, Assisted Living Community; BHC, Behavioral Health Care and Human Services; CAH, Critical Access Hospital; HAP, Hospital; MM, Medication Management; NCC, Nursing Care Center; OBS, Office-Based Surgery Practice; OME, Home Care.

KEY CONCEPT

Safe Storage of Medications

On the most basic level, where and how your organization stores medications are critical to maintaining safety for patients, staff, and visitors. Safe storage also helps preserve the integrity of medications between delivery to the facility and preparation and dispensing to the patient.

Your organization needs to plan to accommodate the safe storage conditions of all medications. Medications should be safely stored according to manufacturers' instructions, which typically provide information on such factors as temperature, humidity, and light conditions. If a medication does not come with storage instructions from the manufacturer, a pharmacist can direct staff on how to safely store it.

The health care and human services fields are vast and provide care, treatment, and services to many individuals who may be referred to as patients, individuals served, residents, consumers, or clients. The term patient *is used throughout this book to describe a recipient of care, treatment, and services.*

Medication Storage Supervision

Joint Commission Medication Management (MM) Standard MM.03.01.01, Element of Performance (EP) 18, requires organizations to periodically inspect all medication storage areas.* Some of the areas of a facility that should be inspected include the pharmacy, floor stock, and automatic dispensing cabinets (ADCs); storage areas for emergency medications kept in patient care areas and sample medications should also be assessed. The inspection should cover the following:

- Proper dating of multidose vials
- Appropriate monitoring and documentation of refrigerator function
- Appropriate response to out-of-range temperature readings
- Secure medication storage facilities and practices
- Cleanliness of the environment
- Assessing for and removing expired medications

Pharmacies at hospitals and critical access hospitals that use Joint Commission accreditation for deemed status with the Centers for Medicare & Medicaid Services (CMS) must be directed by a registered pharmacist or have a supervised medication storage area (see MM.03.01.01, EP 19). In these facilities, the pharmacist or medication storage supervisor should direct periodic inspections and security reviews.

* This is not a requirement for office-based surgery practices.

In all settings, these medication storage inspections are an opportunity to assess how well your organization is adhering to law, regulation, and its policies, as well as how well your policies are serving organizationwide safety and security goals.

Floor Stock

Floor stock is an inventory of medications that are stored in clinical areas outside of the pharmacy for use in that area. Your organization's interdisciplinary medication management team should collaborate to make decisions about which medications will be stored—and how they will be stored—in certain areas, based on the patient population served.

No matter what medications you decide to store in patient care areas, the same need for safe and secure storage applies. You need to devise a storage solution that allows for quick and easy access but that also minimizes variation and potential for error.

Increasingly, organizations are turning to ADCs to store and dispense medications in patient care areas. We'll address ADCs in more detail in Chapter 5 on page 74, but be aware that ADCs are an option for some organizations to help with safe and secure storage and accurate dispensing of medications in patient care areas.

in other words

emergency medication
A medication available for ready use for patient emergencies when dispensing through the pharmacy would not be practical.

floor stock
An inventory of medications that are stored in clinical areas outside of the pharmacy for use in that area.

Emergency Medications

The availability of emergency medications is essential to the operation of hospital emergency departments. But these medications are also critical to patient care and safety throughout the hospital, as well as in treatment and care areas of other health care settings. In short, patients may experience the need for emergent care in a variety of settings and locations, and your organization needs to take steps to ensure that medications needed to provide that care are readily available.

Some hospitals stock commonly used emergency medications in ADCs for easy access and secure storage. In nonhospital settings and smaller hospitals, the use of emergency carts or emergency medication kits is a good way to ensure that common emergency medications are readily available when needed. Those settings whose protocols are to call 911 for emergencies may opt to have certain medications available, such as epinephrine for an allergic reaction, rather than a full emergency medication kit.

When assembling emergency carts or emergency medication kits, consider which medications you are likely to need in an emergency (see sidebar below), as well as which dosages are likely to be required. Even better, emergency medications should be made available in unit-dose, age-specific, and ready-to-administer forms. Also be sure to assess the training and experience of staff members who will be responsible for administering the medications.

Common Emergency Medications

What follows is a basic list of common emergency medications and their uses. If your organization stocks these medications, make sure that they are stocked in doses appropriate to your patient population and that staff members are trained on how to administer them. It's no good to stock medications that require intravenous (IV) administration if no one on hand has training and experience in IV administration.

Common emergency medications and their uses include but are not limited to the following:

- Epinephrine, diphenhydramine, and albuterol for allergic reactions and other respiratory events
- Nitroglycerine for chest pain
- Atropine and ephedrine to combat hypotension and vasovagal syncope
- Glucose for hypoglycemia
- Flumazenil and naloxone to combat opioid overdose and adverse anesthesia events

Assess your need for these and other emergency medications. Consider where to store them so that they will be secure but accessible when needed. These considerations will depend on your patient population, the nature of the care you provide, the physical layout of your facility, and so on. Every practice is different, and Joint Commission standards do not specify how to provide access to emergency medications.

Smart Questions

If the organization stores self-administered medications, can a medical technician or aide remove the medication from storage and hand it, in the container, to the individual to self-administer?

Can a medical technician or aide remove the medication from the container and hand it to the individual?

Can individuals keep medication they brought with them to the facility in their room?

How do individuals report to staff whenever they self-administer medication? How does staff document this?

TRY THIS TOOL

Tool 3-1. Medication Storage and Security Assessment Checklist

This checklist includes questions to ask to assess storage and security of medications in your organization. It can be used to determine if there are risks that need to be mitigated. It can also be used by staff for a daily check.

Medications Brought in by Patients or Their Families

Organizations are required under MM.03.01.05, EP 1, to define whether and when medications brought into the facility by patients can be administered. This includes medications brought in by patients, family members, or prescribers outside the organization for use by patients during their stay.

Such medications must be evaluated by a physician or another qualified staff member to decide whether they should be administered to the patient during his or her time in the facility. To reduce the chances of adverse drug interactions or therapeutic duplication, you'll want to add these medications to the list of medications the patient is taking. In addition, each medication needs to be inspected by a qualified staff member to ensure its integrity.

It is also important to define the role of staff in the administration or self-administration of medications brought in by patients or their families. In some cases, patients may be allowed to keep the medication in their room and self-administer it as needed. In other cases, medications may need to be stored in a more secure location, and staff members may need to deliver the medication to the patient. *See* Chapter 6 on page 87 for details on the requirements of self-administered medications.

KEY CONCEPT

Medication Control

Part of the process of maintaining medication security and safety is devising a system that allows you to track every dose of every medication every step of the way—from the time it is delivered to the organization, through administering the medication to a patient, until the medication and any waste products associated with it are disposed of. Health care organizations that store medications at their facility need a written policy that governs the medication control system, in accordance with MM.03.01.01, EP 4 (see Tool 3-2 on page 41 for a sample policy). The policy must cover the safe and secure storage and handling of every medication, as well as how to dispose of expired or contaminated medications.

This policy is particularly important when it comes to hazardous medications and controlled substances, as state or federal law and regulation may impose special requirements for disposing of these medications. For instance, you may need to have more than one staff member verify the proper disposal of a controlled medication.

Radiopharmaceutical Considerations

For organizations that stock radiopharmaceuticals, special care is required to prevent accidental exposure. Manufacturers' instructions and applicable law and regulation govern the storage and handling of these medications. Furthermore, radiopharmaceuticals must follow the requirements noted in MM standards related to storage, preparation, administration, labeling, and so on. If you are a hospital or critical access hospital that uses Joint Commission accreditation for CMS deemed status, you are required to maintain records of the receipt and disposition of radiopharmaceuticals. These records may be requested by a Joint Commission surveyor, but they can also be used as data for your performance improvement activities.

You should regularly review how well your organization and staff are complying with law, standards, and your own organization's policies regarding the handling and use of radiopharmaceuticals. These reviews can help in a number of ways, including assessing adherence to law, regulation, and United States Pharmacopeia guidelines (*see* page 15 in Chapter 1); guiding performance improvement activities; and improving survey readiness.

Secure Storage

Controlled medications, such as opioids, stimulants, and depressants, are used in a variety of health care contexts. It can be challenging to keep these medications secure (in accordance with Standard MM.03.01.01, EP 3) and track them in all types of situations (MM.05.01.11, EP 2). However, ensuring that all medications and biologicals, including controlled medications, are secured is required.

In many health care organizations, secure storage involves storing controlled substances in locked cabinets, among other measures. This may not be practical in all settings, however. For instance, in home care and community-based behavioral health care and human services settings, you may not have access to a locking

in other words

controlled medication
A drug or other substance that is tightly controlled by the government because of its potential for abuse or addiction.

medication control
The tracking and documentation of the movement of medication from the time it enters the facility until it is administered and/or disposed of.

radiopharmaceuticals
Radioactive compounds used for diagnostic or therapeutic purposes.

TRY THIS TOOL

Tool 3-2. Medication Control Policy

This sample medication control policy features elements to consider including in a policy for your organization. Be sure to customize the sample to suit the needs and requirements of your organization.

cabinet. You should consult with a pharmacist and refer to federal regulations to develop ideas for securing controlled substances in such situations.

Collaboration

The decision-making process for how to store bedside medications is an opportunity for cross-disciplinary collaboration. Organization leadership can conduct a proactive risk assessment for each situation under consideration. Inform this risk assessment with data, experience, and expertise provided by pharmacists, nurses, prescribers, building engineers, environment of care professionals, and others.

Your bedside medication storage policy may cover so many different medications that a one-size-fits-all solution is not workable. Leadership can help guide thinking on how to allocate staff and resources efficiently to achieve your medication safety and security goals. As always, the final pieces of this puzzle include a system for monitoring how well the policy works, a mechanism for reporting problems, and a plan for how to address them. Leadership also has a role here in ensuring that staff buy into a culture of safety and continuous performance improvement.

Medication Access

Another key part of medication control is limiting who has access to medications. Study the laws and regulations that address who can have access to certain medications, and become familiar with your organization's responsibilities in this area, particularly when dealing with controlled substances. Your state's board of pharmacy can assist with this process.

Your organization should already have a broad policy that governs who can access the pharmacy, medication safes, locked cabinets containing medications, and so on. You may choose to divide staff members into categories, according to their access privileges, or to keep lists of staff members who are authorized to access medication storage areas or handle specific medications.

Medication Security in Home Care

In home care settings, medication storage and supervision standards apply only to organizations that store medications on site. Furthermore, inpatient hospices that use Joint Commission accreditation for CMS deemed status must abide by some specific rules. These special requirements, detailed below, represent added layers of caution and security that other organizations may consider including in their own policies.

- The hospice must maintain records of the receipt and disposition of all controlled medications to facilitate medication reconciliation.
- The organization must audit the hospice's controlled medication records for accuracy and reconciliation.
- The hospice must store controlled medications in a locked compartment in accordance with state and federal laws. The only personnel who have access to the locked compartment are those who are authorized to do so.
- The pharmacist and the hospice administrator immediately investigate discrepancies that occur at any point in the process of procuring, storing, dispensing, administering, disposing of, or returning controlled medications.
- The organization must immediately report to the appropriate state authority discrepancies that occur at any point in the process of procuring, storing, dispensing, administering, disposing of, or returning controlled medications. The organization must conduct a thorough investigation of any discrepancies and provide a written report of the investigation to state and federal officials, when required by law or regulation.

KEY CONCEPT

Managing Medications in the Inventory

Medications that are expired, damaged, or contaminated pose an elevated risk of patient harm. Your organization will need to create a process for periodically reviewing your inventory to identify such medications. You might consider adding checks for damage, expiration, or contamination into your dispensing and administration protocols.

When a medication is identified as expired, damaged, or contaminated, staff should immediately remove it from circulation and return it to the location specified by organization policy, where the medication can be properly processed and disposed of. The protocols for removing and storing expired, damaged, or contaminated medications may be subject to law and regulation, particularly in the case of controlled substances. Be sure to also include documentation procedures in your protocols.

Retrieving Recalled Medications

The risk to patients of recalled medications really can't be overstated. If a medication is recalled by the manufacturer or the US Food and Drug Administration (FDA) for safety reasons, your organization will need to inform the prescribers of that medication and anyone involved in the dispensing or administration of the medication. A robust medication control policy and system should help you quickly identify where all quantities of a given medication are within your organization. Do this quickly to stop any more of the medication from being dispensed or administered. Administering recalled medication may put patients at risk for adverse drug events and expose the organization and/or staff to liability.

in other words

recalled medication

Medication that is removed from circulation for safety reasons by the manufacturer, the FDA, or another agency.

After the recalled medication is collected, you must dispose of it according to manufacturer's instruction and/or law and regulation. In some cases, you may need to return the medication to the manufacturer.

The Joint Commission requires a written policy that describes what steps your organization and individual staff will take to retrieve and handle doses or quantities of the recalled medication that you have on hand (in accordance with MM.05.01.17, EP 1).* Your policy should contain specific answers to these and other questions:

- Which patients are affected?
- Who will receive recall notifications?
- Who else will need to be informed of the recall?
- What happens next?

TRY THIS TOOL

Tool 3-3. Recalled Medication Management Policy

This sample policy can help you determine the steps your organization should take in the event of a medication recall. Be sure to adapt the sample to meet the specific needs and requirements of your organization.

Your policy, law, regulation, or the terms of the medication recall may require you to inform patients about it. If so, work with your organization's legal counsel and/or risk manager to determine the best course of action. Recalls may be alarming to patients, so keep it simple, direct, and transparent. Let the patient know the name

* This is not a requirement for assisted living communities.

of the recalled medication, the reasons for the recall, what steps the organization is taking to ensure patient safety, and applicable rights the patient has to additional information and resources.

Returning Expired, Damaged, or Recalled Medications

Medication that is expired or otherwise returned to the pharmacy needs to be accounted for, controlled, and/or properly disposed of by your organization to promote patient safety. Develop a process for doing this that covers what medications can be returned, what the return process looks like, and how you will document it.

In some circumstances, your organization may contract with an outside entity to dispose of expired, damaged, or recalled medications. Document this process as well, including what medications are covered in the contract, and the process for collecting and transferring them to the contractor. Certain aspects of the return and disposal of medications, particularly high-alert medications and controlled substances, may be covered by law or regulation. Familiarize yourself with applicable laws and rules.

With so many aspects of safe and secure storage of medications governed by Joint Commission standards, law, regulation, and manufacturers' instructions, you might feel overwhelmed. But these different structures represent interlocking and complementary frameworks to help you keep your medications safely and securely stored. As always, The Joint Commission and appropriate government agencies can help you interpret standards, laws, and regulations in the context of your organization and setting.

Additional Resources

- United States Pharmacopeia (USP) is an independent scientific nonprofit organization that works to ensure the safety, efficacy, and availability of pharmaceutical products. https://www.usp.org/

Smart Questions

How will you alert applicable staff in your organization about medication recalls?

Who is responsible for notifying prescribers?

How will you notify prescribers?

Under what circumstances will you inform the patient?

CHAPTER 4

Ordering and Transcribing Medications

The point in the medication management system at which staff communicates and transcribes medication orders is one of the major risk points. Your organization is responsible for training staff on the ordering and transcription process to avoid confusion, misunderstanding, and errors related to medications.

It is also important to have organization policies and procedures in place to help reduce the probability of error and variation. These policies should cover various aspects of the ordering and transcribing process, including the types of acceptable orders, the components of valid orders, how to handle titration orders, and what to do when an order is incomplete, illegible, unclear, or invalid. This chapter will address these processes in more detail.

KEY CONCEPTS

- Communicating Medication Orders
- Medication Order Types
- Look-Alike/Sound-Alike Medications
- High-Alert and Hazardous Medications

The Standards

Following are the relevant standards for the content in this chapter from your setting's *Comprehensive Accreditation Manual* or its E-dition® counterpart.

Standard	AHC	ALC	BHC	CAH	HAP	NCC	OBS	OME
EC.02.02.01 The [organization] manages risks related to hazardous materials and waste.	X	X	X	X	X	X	X	X
MM.01.01.01 The [organization] plans its medication management processes.	X	X	X	X	X	X	X	X
MM.01.01.03 The [organization] safely manages high-alert and hazardous medications.	X	X	X	X	X	X	X	X
MM.01.02.01 The [organization] addresses the safe use of look-alike/ sound-alike medications.	X	X	X	X	X	X	X	X
MM.04.01.01 Medication orders are clear and accurate.	X	X	X	X	X	X	X	X
PC.02.01.03 The [organization] provides care, treatment, and services [as ordered or prescribed, and in accordance with law and regulation].	X	X	X*	X	X	X	X	X
RC.02.03.07 Qualified staff receive and record verbal orders.	X	X	X	X	X	X	X	X

AHC: Ambulatory Health Care; BHC: Behavioral Health Care and Human Services; CAH: Critical Access Hospital; HAP: EC, Environment of Care; Hospital; MM, Medication Management; NCC: Nursing Care Center; OBS: Office-Based Surgery Practice; OME: Home Care; PC, Provision of Care, Treatment, and Services; RC, Record of Care, Treatment, and Services.

* This requirement is addressed in Care, Treatment, and Services (CTS) Standard CTS.03.01.03.

KEY CONCEPT

Communicating Medication Orders

Developing a written policy that defines all the required elements of a complete medication order is the most effective way for your organization to ensure clear, complete orders and reduce variation. In fact, Joint Commission Medication Management (MM) Standard MM.04.01.01, Element of Performance (EP) 2, requires such a written policy, with the following minimum requirements of a complete order included in it:

- Medication name
- Medication dose
- Medication route
- Medication frequency

Your medication order policy should also define when the order requires an indication for use, as with orders for medications to be administered as needed (PRN orders), as well as include precautions for ordering potential look-alike/sound-alike medications. We'll discuss precautions and policies associated with look-alike/sound-alike medications later in this chapter (see page 67). For now, what you need to know is that orders for such medications may require additional information, such as the medication brand name in addition to the generic name.

The medication order policy also needs to contain clear instructions for what to do if an order is incomplete, illegible, or unclear. The process should include instructions for clarifying or completing the order, as well as what to do if the person who submitted the order cannot be reached.

Verbal Orders and Preprinted Forms

If possible, you should discourage verbal medication orders. Verbal orders are more prone to variation through misspeaking or mishearing than written or electronic orders. In fact, many organizations prohibit verbal orders outright. Others may allow them only in certain well-defined circumstances, and they often require a written follow-up order within a specified time frame. Home care organizations, for example, take verbal, phone, fax, and electronic media orders more often than other kinds of organizations. However, in some home care settings, physicians are required to communicate verbal orders only to a licensed nurse, nurse practitioner, pharmacist, or other physician.

TRY THIS TOOL

Tool 4-1. Medication Orders Policy

Use this sample medication orders policy to help you understand the required elements as you develop your own policy. Be sure to adapt the sample to suit the needs and requirements of your organization.

Smart Questions

What are the basic required elements of a medication order?

in other words

medication dose
The amount of medication to be administered to the patient per dose or per unit of time (for example, milligrams/hour).

medication frequency
How often medication is to be administered.

medication route
The path by which medication is introduced into the body.

PRN medications
Medications that are provided to the patient to be taken "as needed."

picture this

Figure 4-1. Complete Medication Orders

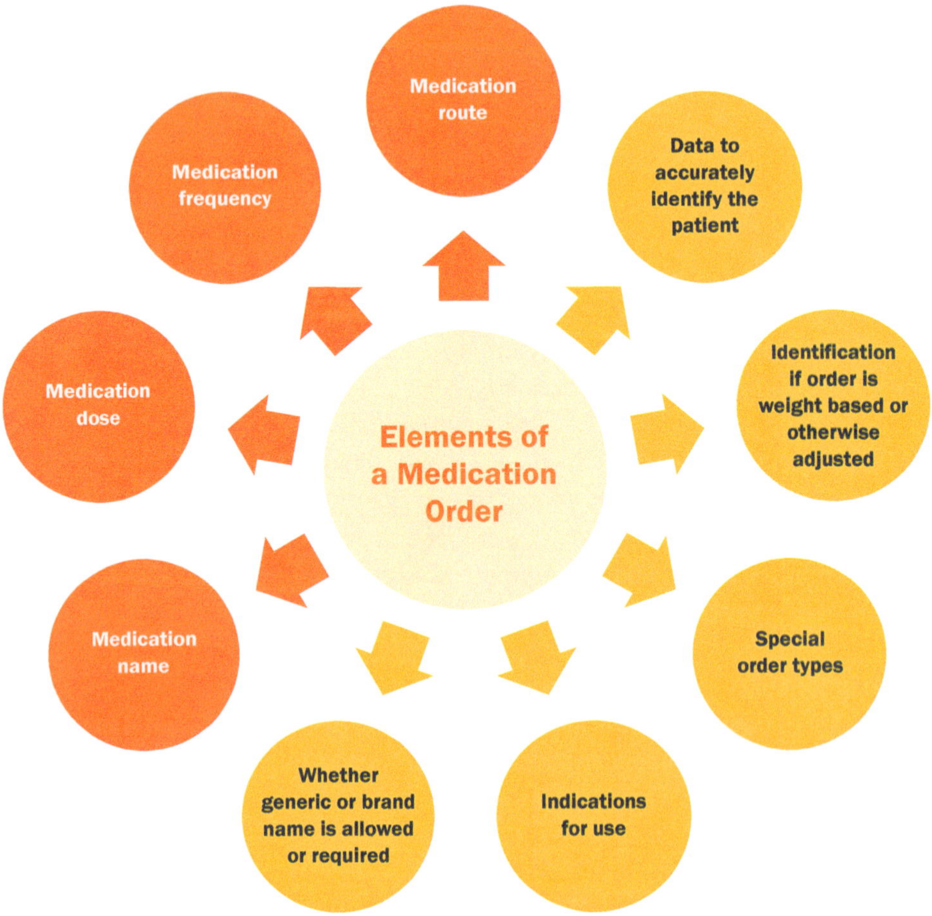

Completeness is essential for all medication orders and prescriptions. This graphic shows the minimum elements of a complete order in orange, as well as some other useful elements you may choose to include in yellow. Your organization can define which elements it will require beyond these. Of course, not all elements will apply to each order; however, you should define which elements apply to which medications.

Prohibited Abbreviations

The use of abbreviations is a common time-saving practice in medication ordering, but some abbreviations can be confusing and increase the likelihood of an error. Below is a list of prohibited abbreviations assembled by The Joint Commission that applies to all orders and all medication-related documentation that is handwritten (including free-text computer entry) or on preprinted forms. You can monitor the medication ordering process to identify and eliminate other problematic abbreviations. Electronic ordering and transcription systems can help eliminate the use of such abbreviations as well.

Do Not Use	Potential Problem	Use Instead
U, u (unit)	Mistaken for "0" (zero), the number "4" (four), or "cc"	Write "unit"
IU (international unit)	Mistaken for IV (intravenous) or the number "10" (ten)	Write "International Unit"
Q.D., QD, q.d., qd (daily) Q.O.D., QOD, q.o.d., qod (every other day)	Mistaken for each other Period after the "Q" mistaken for "I" and the "O" mistaken for "I"	Write "daily" Write "every other day"
Trailing zero (X.0 mg)* Lack of leading zero (.X mg)	Decimal point is missed	Write "X mg" Write "0.X mg"
MS MSO_4 and $MgSO_4$	Can mean morphine sulfate or magnesium sulfate Confused for one another	Write "morphine sulfate" Write "magnesium sulfate"

* A "trailing zero" may be used only where required to demonstrate the level of precision of the value being reported, such as for laboratory results, imaging studies that report size of lesions, or catheter/tube sizes. It may not be used in medication orders or other medication-related documentation.

Given the specific circumstances of your organization and operations, it may not be practical to eliminate all verbal and/or phone orders from your practice. If your organization chooses to allow verbal orders, such orders should be documented thoroughly according to organization policy and Joint Commission Record of Care, Treatment, and Services (RC) Standard RC.02.03.07. Documentation must include the date and time of the order and the names and roles of everyone involved: who placed the order, who received the order, who recorded the order, and who implemented the order. Before taking action on the verbal order, staff must use a record and "read back" process to verify the information, according to Provision of Care, Treatment, and Services (PC) Standard PC.02.01.03, EP 20.

You might consider also using preprinted order sheets or electronic order sets. These forms will decrease miscommunication, misinterpretation, transcription errors, and other variations, and they encourage medication order completeness. If you do choose to use preprinted forms, Joint Commission Standard MM.04.01.01, EP 7, requires that you review and update the forms periodically and whenever problems arise. Make your updates according to current evidence and practices.

Smart Questions

Whom should you contact to clear up or complete a medication order? How do you initiate that discussion?

What do you do if the person who submitted the order cannot be reached?

What safety precautions do you require for verbal or phone orders?

Medication Order Errors

To err is human—and common. Some of the most common causes of medication errors include the following:

- Poor communication (incomplete patient information, miscommunication of medication orders)
- Confusion in product names, dosing units, and medical abbreviations
- Incorrect labeling
- Care recipient's misunderstanding directions for medication use

A large percentage of medication errors occur when new orders are written during the admission or discharge of a care recipient. Of course, incomplete, illegible, or unclear orders at any point along the care continuum can lead to medication errors. That's why all medication orders must be clear and accurate—wherever and whenever medications are ordered, dispensed, and administered. The idea is to curtail confusion and eliminate errors.

PRN (as needed) medication orders can create confusion because there are typically several orders written for the same purpose—without clarification about when one medication should be given versus another. Verbal orders can cause confusion too, so qualified individuals must authenticate any verbal medication order with a read-back procedure for verification. Verbal orders (including telephone orders) should be kept to a minimum, and texting orders are prohibited.

Medication Order Errors (continued)

So how do you ensure that medication orders are complete, clear, and accurate? Here are just a few areas to focus on:

- **Review documents.** Review your organization policy on medication orders and make sure it includes everything required by Joint Commission standards, as well as law and regulation for your specific setting.
- **Conduct tracers.** Perform regular audits of medication orders as part of your mock tracers to assess for sustained organization policy and standards compliance.
- **Provide education.** Along with the audits, educate staff on how to respond to noncompliant medication orders per your policy. You might want to provide them with a brief script they could use when calling prescribers to clarify an order.
- **Facilitate processes.** Review preprinted orders and order sets to ensure that they support safe prescribing. Work with staff and providers to get ideas on how orders can be improved.
- **Encourage technology use.** Required elements of medication orders can be built into a computerized provider order entry (CPOE) system for increased assurance.

At a basic level, every complete medication order is based on a diagnosis, a condition, or an indication for use. This information doesn't need to appear on each medication order, but it must be written somewhere, such as in the patient's medical or clinical record. Making this information available helps improve understanding between staff and licensed independent practitioners involved in the medication management process.

in other words

tracer methodology

A process surveyors use during the survey to analyze an organization's systems or processes for delivering safe, high-quality care by following an individual patient or resident through the organization's care process in the sequence experienced by each individual. Depending on the setting, this process may require surveyors to visit multiple care programs and services within an organization or within a single program or service to "trace" the care rendered.

Smart Questions

As a licensed independent practitioner or staff member who participates in the management of a patient's medications, where can you find relevant information about the patient? How will you access this information?

Minimum Basic Patient Information

In most settings, Joint Commission Standard MM.01.01.01, EP 1, requires organizations to have a written policy describing how important, basic patient information will be made available to those involved in the patient's care and management of his or her medications. Your organization's policy should identify essential information to include, such as the following:

- Age
- Sex
- Diagnoses
- Allergies
- Sensitivities
- Current medications
- Height and weight
- Pregnancy and lactation information (when applicable)
- Laboratory results (when applicable)
- Any additional information required by the organization

The requirements vary across settings. For example, nursing care centers are not required to have a written policy stating how this information is made available, but they are still responsible for making sure it is made available to those who participate in the management of patients' medications.

If you work in a hospital or critical access hospital, or a behavioral health care and human services organization that prescribes medications, you not only must have a written policy covering how the above information is made available to staff, but, according to Leadership (LD) standards, you also need to facilitate practitioners' access to the prescription drug monitoring program (PDMP) database. The PDMP is a program run at the state level and overseen by the Centers for Disease Control and Prevention (CDC) to help track the prescription and distribution of opioid medications and other controlled substances (*see* https://www.cdc.gov/drugoverdose/pdmp/providers.html for PDMP provider information).

KEY CONCEPT

Medication Order Types

Each organization must develop a written policy listing the types of medication orders that are acceptable for use. Based on your organization's setting, patient population, size, capabilities, and other factors, you will determine what kinds of orders you will allow and make sure that all staff involved in medication management knows what types of orders are acceptable. Your policy also must detail what the required minimum elements are for each type of order.

Commonly used types of orders include the following:

Order Type	Description
As needed (PRN) orders	Orders acted on based on the occurrence of a specific indication or symptom
Automatic stop orders	Orders that include a date or time to discontinue a medication
Compounding orders	Orders for compounded drugs or drug mixtures not commercially available
Device orders	Orders for medication-related devices, such as nebulizers, catheters, or other devices
Discharge orders	Orders for medications to be given to the patient at discharge or transfer
Herbal orders	Orders for herbal products
Investigational medication orders	Orders for medications involved in research protocols or clinical trials
Range orders	Orders in which the dose or dosing interval varies over a prescribed range, depending on the situation or the patient's status
Signed and held orders	New prewritten (held) medication orders and specific instructions from a licensed independent practitioner to administer medication(s) to a patient in clearly defined circumstances that become active upon the release of the orders on a specific date(s) and time(s)
Standing orders	Prewritten medication orders with specific instructions from a licensed independent practitioner to administer a medication to a person in clearly defined circumstances

Order Type	Description
Taper orders	Orders in which the dose is decreased by a particular amount each dosing interval
Titration orders	Orders in which the dose is progressively increased or decreased in response to a patient's status

Summary Orders

When a patient is admitted to a facility, sometimes the care team stops any medications currently being taken to assess the patient's condition and reduce the probability of adverse drug interactions. There may be other situations in which a patient's normal medication may be suspended for a time. Because of the elevated risk of patient harm summary (blanket) orders pose, Joint Commission Standard MM.04.01.01, EP 8,* requires organizations that prescribe medications to prohibit summary orders for the resumption of previous medications. This will not only mitigate the risk of adverse events, but it also will encourage a full review of the medications a patient is taking and the reasons for each, including an assessment of the benefits, risks, and utility of each medication.

TRY THIS TOOL

Tool 4-2. Mock Tracer Worksheet: Medication Ordering

Use this worksheet to conduct mock tracers with your staff. It can help you identify weak areas in your medication ordering process.

Collaboration

Your organization's medical staff, nursing staff, and pharmacy leadership need to work together on a periodic review of any standing orders, order sets, and protocols for medication orders. These reviews should include an examination of standing orders and protocols for consistency with nationally recognized and evidence-based guidelines, as well as a review to assess their continuing usefulness and safety.

in other words

titration orders

Orders in which the dose may be increased or decreased in response to changes in the patient's status. Titration is a way to limit potential side effects by taking time to see how the patient reacts to a medication.

Titration Orders

Titration orders are medication orders for which the dosage is increased or decreased by a nurse in response to the patient's status. This applies not just to medication infusions but also to oral, topical, injectable, and other medication orders in which the dosage may be adjusted in this way. Staff should take special

* This is not a requirement for assisted living communities.

care when communicating and transcribing titration orders because the number of variables increases the risk of harm to the patient through medication error.

For this reason, Joint Commission Standard MM.04.01.01, EP 2, requires that, when applicable, an organization's medication orders policy must define the special rules governing titration orders. Titration orders must include the following:

- Medication name
- Medication route
- Initial rate of infusion, if applicable (dose/unit of time)
- Incremental units to which the rate or dose can be increased or decreased
- How often you can change the rate or dose
- Maximum rate or dose of infusion
- Objective clinical measures staff will use to guide changes

Some organizations may choose to have a medication titration orders policy separate from their medication orders policy (see Tool 4-4). Consider the use of special preprinted order sheets for titration orders, and make sure that each order contains clear instructions for how and when to adjust the titration.

KEY CONCEPT

Look-Alike/Sound-Alike Medications

At a time when so many medications are available, it's not surprising that some have similarly spelled names, names that sound like the names of others, or names that visually look similar to each other. This is an obvious area of potential confusion and could lead to the wrong medication being given to a patient. However, you can put safeguards in place to prevent this kind of critical error by developing sound strategies to address look-alike/sound-alike medications.

Look-Alike/Sound-Alike Medications List

To protect your patients from errors related to look-alike/sound-alike medications, begin by creating a list of all the potential look-alike/sound-alike medications your organization stores, dispenses, or administers. The Institute for Safe Medication Practices (ISMP) identifies commonly confused medications on its website (see https://www.ismp.org/recommendations/confused-drug-names-list). This list will get you started. Include brand names and generic names in one column and suggested

Smart Questions

What information is required for a titration order?

Do you have special forms for titration orders that are specifically designed for those orders?

Is it feasible to create separate forms in an electronic ordering system for each order type?

TRY THIS TOOL

Tool 4-3. Sample Titration Order Form

Use this tool to develop a titration order form designed to prevent communication and transcription errors in the ordering process. Be sure to adapt this sample form to meet the needs and requirements of your organization.

Tool 4-4. Medication Titration Orders Policy

Use this sample policy to develop a medication titration order policy that increases clarity, reduces variation, and works for your organization.

in other **words**

look-alike/sound-alike medications
Pairs or larger groups of medications that have sufficiently similar names that they present an elevated risk of confusing one with another.

actions to mitigate risk of error in another column (see Figure 4-2 on page 59 for an example). The medication names may not begin with similarly spelled or sounding names; sometimes it is how the name ends that may cause confusion (for example, ALPRAZolam, LORazepam, and clonazepam).

Your organization should have a formulary that lists all the medications available to prescribe, along with strength and dosage information (see "Creating and Maintaining a Formulary" in Chapter 2 on page 29). Review your formulary and see if you can spot other potentially confusing pairs. Have any medication errors occurred as a result of confusion when one medication was intended and another similar-sounding one was selected? Add these to your list. Don't forget to include sample medications.

When you have populated this list, make sure it's available to anyone involved in the medication management process by posting it where medication management activities take place, including in or on the following areas:

- Medication rooms
- Patient homes or residential living areas
- Infirmaries
- Crash carts
- Automatic dispensing cabinets
- Dental carts
- Bulk storage medication cabinets
- Narcotics locked storage cabinets
- Anesthesia carts
- Block carts
- Treatment rooms
- Immunization rooms

Smart Questions

What extra precautions are required for ordering look-alike/sound-alike medications?

Special Precautions

To reduce the potential for error related to look-alike/sound-alike medications, take steps to ensure that medication orders are clear and the correct medication is administered. For instance, in some cases you might include both the brand name and the generic name of the medication in the order. As an alternative, you could include the purpose of the medication in the prescription.

Changing the appearance of the names of commonly confused medications on labels is another option. For example, capitalizing the portions of medication names that differ from their commonly confused counterparts (using tall man lettering) can help alert staff

picture this

Figure 4-2. Look-Alike/Sound-Alike Medications Worksheet

Look-Alike/Sound-Alike Medications	Suggested Actions
cloNIDine (Catapres®) Klonopin® (clonazePAM)	• Separate products stored in pharmacy. • Affix auxiliary label on storage bin to heighten staff awareness. • Use tall man characters to alert prescriber and nursing staff when they access Pyxis machine.
PACLitaxel (Taxol®) DOCEtaxel (Taxotere®)	• Do not accept verbal orders. • Install maximum dose warning for each drug in the computer. • Label shelf with colored label and "look-alike/sound-alike" identifier. • Double-check pharmacy process prior to dispensing. • Check product against order before leaving the pharmacy and prior to administration.

This is just a sample of what a Look-Alike/Sound-Alike Medications Worksheet might look like, with a few sample entries filled in. Your list would obviously be much longer and contain many more medications.

to the potential for a mixup. The US Food and Drug Administration (FDA) and ISMP both provide recommendations on how to do this, including ISMP's list of commonly confused medication names and recommended tall man capitalization forms (see https://www.ismp.org/recommendations/tall-man-letters-list).

Another way your organization might reduce variation and risk of error with look-alike/sound-alike medications is to build alerts into electronic ordering and record systems for specific drugs that could be potentially confused with a look-alike/sound-alike medication. It is also wise to avoid having look-alike/sound-alike pairs from appearing consecutively in lists and menus or storing them next to each other.

Have your medication management team review the look-alike/sound-alike list at least once per year or more often if your organization frequently adds medications to its formulary. The review is an opportunity for people involved in all aspects of medication management to update the list based on new

picture this

Figure 4-3. Examples of Look-Alike/Sound-Alike Medications

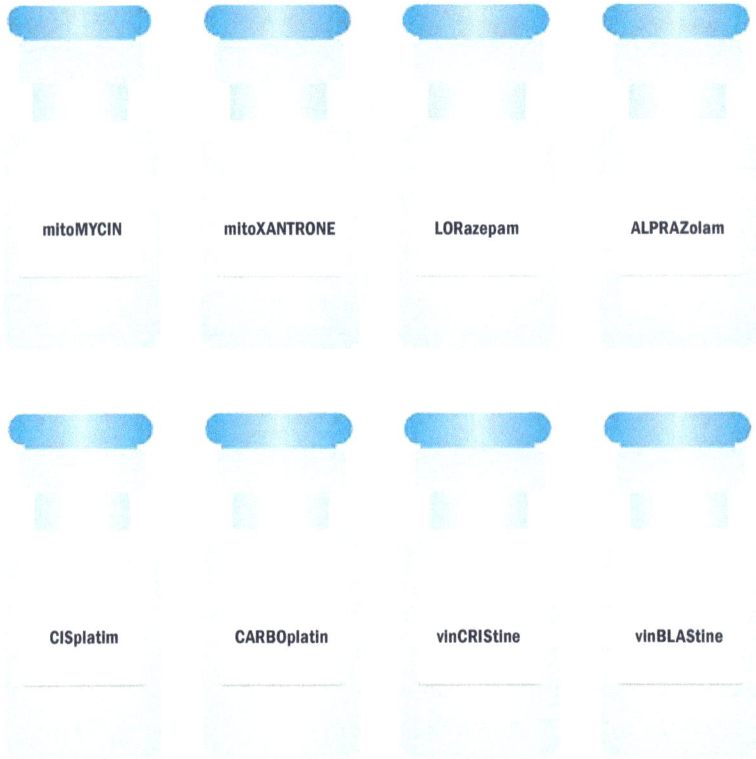

Tall man lettering on labels, such as those shown above, can be very helpful in look-alike/sound-alike medication pairs.

recommendations from ISMP, as well as to suggest new pairs or trios for the list and new ways of reducing confusion.

KEY CONCEPT

High-Alert and Hazardous Medications

Another risk area for your medication management team to address is high-alert and hazardous medications. High-alert medications are those that could be particularly harmful to patients if they are used in error. These include opioids, insulin, anticoagulants, and others that present a higher risk of causing a sentinel event or other significant adverse drug event. Devote special care and planning to all aspects of management of high-alert medications.

Likewise, pay careful attention to hazardous medications in your formulary. Studies in animals and humans indicate that exposure to hazardous medications can cause cancer, developmental or reproductive toxicity, genotoxicity, or harm to organs. If not properly handled, they can pose a risk to patients and staff. And because these medications can become part of the physical environment via spills and leaks, The Joint Commission also discusses them in the "Environment of Care" (EC) chapter's hazardous materials and waste standard, EC.02.02.01, EP 8 (in addition to Standard MM.01.01.03).

Joint Commission Standard MM.01.01.03, EP 1 requires organizations to identify, in writing, their high-alert and hazardous medications. ISMP maintains a list of high-alert medications for acute care, long term care, and ambulatory care settings in its resource library (see https://www.ismp.org/recommendations). The National Institute for Occupational Safety and Health (NIOSH) also keeps a list of hazardous medications you may consult (see https://www.cdc.gov/niosh/docs/2016-161/pdfs/2016-161.pdf?id=10.26616/NIOSHPUB2016161). Both organizations periodically update the information, but you should also develop your list by reviewing your formulary. Consider usage patterns, error data, risk analysis, and safety issues reported in the literature in your assessment. All hazardous medications used in your organization that appear on the ISMP and NIOSH lists must be included on your list.

Depending on your setting and circumstances, you may also choose to include sample medications, investigational medications,

TRY THIS TOOL

Tool 4-5. Look-Alike/Sound-Alike Medication Management Policy Development Checklist

This checklist is designed to help you create or improve your look-alike/sound-alike medication management policy.

psychotherapeutic medications, and controlled substances. Some of the medications on your list will come with handling, storage, and dispensing rules that are a matter of regulation or law.

After this list is created, Joint Commission standards require a process for managing high-alert and hazardous medications. Following are just a few steps you could take to stay on top of this task:

- **Collaborate with experts.** Schedule regular meetings among or with pharmacists to keep up to date on the required formulary lists for high-alert medications and hazardous medications stocked by your organization. Talk about the processes to mitigate risks within each category. Work with environment of care staff on disposal of any hazardous medications.
- **Provide education.** Pull together high-alert and hazardous medications resources available from ISMP, the Occupational Safety and Health Administration (OSHA), and NIOSH. Make them available in one place for all staff to reference.
- **Conduct tracers.** Make high-alert and hazardous medications a periodic focus for system tracers in relevant areas of your organization.
- **Track errors and variations.** Such tracking can be an integral part of your performance improvement activities.

TRY THIS TOOL

Tool 4-6. High-Alert and Hazardous Medication Management Policy

Use this sample policy to help you develop or adapt a high-alert and hazardous medications policy. Be sure to customize it to meet your organization's needs and requirements.

Smart Questions

What strategies do you have in place to manage high-risk, hazardous, and look-alike/ sound-alike medications?

in other words

high-alert medication

High-alert medications are drugs that bear a heightened risk of causing significant patient harm when they are used in error.

hazardous medication

A medication in which studies in animals or humans indicate that exposure to them has a potential for causing cancer, developmental or reproductive toxicity, genotoxicity, or harm to organs.

Collaboration

Joint Commission standards require nursing care organizations that prescribe psychotropic medications to come up with and implement an interdisciplinary monitoring system, including the physician, pharmacist, nursing staff, and others involved in the care team. This team can monitor patients for side effects, evaluate the effects and efficacy of the medication, watch out for errors or other adverse events, and collect data on the use of psychotropic medications by the organization. These data can inform your medication management and performance improvement activities. As such, although The Joint Commission does not require this kind of interdisciplinary monitoring in other settings, it is a good idea, particularly when it comes to psychotropic medications.

Special Requirements for Controlled Substances in Certain Settings

Some organizations choose to include controlled substances on their list of high-alert medications. Depending on your health care setting, there may be special handling or reporting requirements related to controlled substances. For instance, Joint Commission standards require hospitals using Joint Commission accreditation for deemed status with the Centers for Medicare & Medicaid Services (CMS) to ensure that any abuse or loss of controlled substances be reported to the person who manages the pharmacy, and in some cases to the chief executive.

Psychotropic medications may play a larger role in treatment in certain kinds of nursing care facilities, such as memory support or dementia units, and some behavioral health care and human services organizations. Joint Commission standards for behavioral health care and human services organizations require a written policy that addresses the use of multiple psychotropic agents in the same class; the use of high-dose pharmacotherapy; and the prevention, identification, and management of side effects.

In nursing care centers, clinicians may prescribe psychotropic medications when indicated by assessment and medical necessity, but only after considering or trying other nonpharmacological interventions or alternatives—and at the lowest effective therapeutic dose. Develop a system to monitor the use of these medications and review the system periodically to see if the management and monitoring systems are producing the desired outcomes. Particularly when prescribing antipsychotic medications, nursing care centers must closely monitor their use and involve patients (to the extent possible), or their family or legal representative, in the decision to use antipsychotic medication. Any patient admitted on an antipsychotic medication must have his or her case reviewed by the attending physician and consulting pharmacist to determine if the medication is appropriate and necessary, if the dosage might be reduced, or if there might be other alternatives. Provide education about the use, benefits, and risks of psychotropic medications as part of the required patient and family education given to dementia patients and their families.

in other words

psychotropic medication

A medication that affects the central nervous system and that is prescribed with the intention of affecting psychological processes such as perception, mental status, or behavior. Examples of classes of psychotropic medications include antipsychotics, antidepressants, anxiolytics, hypnotics, and sedatives.

The processes of ordering and transcribing medication orders present significant potential for miscommunication and confusion. Sound policies governing the components of different kinds of orders, how they are communicated, and how issues are resolved can help significantly reduce the probability of errors. The adoption of digital ordering and pharmacy information systems can also help increase clarity and completeness of orders and should be seriously considered by your medication management team.

Additional Resources

- The Institute for Safe Medication Practices (ISMP) has a list (https://www.ismp.org/recommendations/confused-drug-names-list) of commonly confused medication names on its website. The organization also offers a list (https://www.ismp.org/recommendations/tall-man-letters-list) of look-alike medication names with tall man letters. For information on high-alert medications, see ISMP's lists for ambulatory care (https://www.ismp.org/recommendations/high-alert-medications-community-ambulatory-list), long term care (https://www.ismp.org/recommendations/high-alert-medications-long-term-care-list), and acute care (https://www.ismp.org/recommendations/high-alert-medications-acute-list) settings.
- The National Institute for Occupational Safety and Health (NIOSH) maintains a list of hazardous medications. https://www.cdc.gov/niosh/docs/2016-161/default.html
- Prescription Drug Monitoring Programs (PDMPs) are overseen by the Centers for Disease Control and Prevention (CDC) to help track the prescription and distribution of opioid medications and other controlled substances. https://www.cdc.gov/drugoverdose/pdmp/providers.html

CHAPTER 5

Preparing and Dispensing Medications

When a medication order is received in the pharmacy, the pharmacist and pharmacy staff begin the process of reviewing the order, preparing the medication, ensuring that the medication is properly labeled, and dispensing the medication to the authorized person. The pharmacist is also responsible for devising a policy and system that allow staff to obtain needed medications during times when the pharmacy may be closed or a pharmacist is unavailable.

Please note that the review, preparation, and dispensing processes may be subject to federal and state law and regulation. Familiarize yourself with applicable law, and use that knowledge to inform your policies and procedures related to medication preparation and dispensing.

KEY CONCEPTS

- Reviewing Medication Orders
- Safe Preparation of Medication Orders
- Labeling Medications
- Dispensing Medications
- Obtaining Medications

The Standards

Following are the relevant standards for the content in this chapter from your setting's *Comprehensive Accreditation Manual* or its E-dition® counterpart.

Standard	AHC	ALC	BHC	CAH	HAP	NCC	OBS	OME
MM.05.01.01 [A pharmacist] reviews the appropriateness of all medication orders for medications to be dispensed in the [organization].	X		X	X	X	X	X	X
MM.05.01.07 The [organization] safely prepares medications.	X	X	X	X	X	X	X	X
MM.05.01.09 Medications are labeled.	X	X	X	X	X	X	X	X
MM.05.01.11 The [organization] safely dispenses medications.	X		X	X	X		X	X
MM.05.01.13 The [organization] safely obtains medications when the pharmacy is closed.			X	X	X			X
MM.08.01.01 The [organization] evaluates the effectiveness of its medication management system.	X	X	X	X	X	X	X	X
NPSG.03.04.01 Label all medications, medication containers, and other solutions on and off the sterile field in perioperative and other procedural settings.	X			X	X		X	

AHC, Ambulatory Health Care; ALC, Assisted Living Community; BHC, Behavioral Health Care and Human Services; CAH, Critical Access Hospital; HAP, Hospital; MM, Medication Management; NCC, Nursing Care Center; NPSG, National Patient Safety Goals; OBS, Office-Based Surgery Practice; OME, Home Care.

KEY CONCEPT

Reviewing Medication Orders

All medication orders must be reviewed to make sure they are appropriate. In facilities where the pharmacy is not open 24 hours a day, 7 days a week, your organization can designate a qualified individual to review orders, but the pharmacist will need to perform an additional review when the pharmacy reopens. After the order has been reviewed, all concerns, issues, or questions must be clarified with the prescriber before the medication can be dispensed.

The review process is a critical quality control step. The pharmacist checks each medication order against patient records for the following:

- Patient allergies or potential sensitivities
- Possible interactions with a patient's current medications
- Appropriateness of medication, dose, frequency, and route
- Current or potential impact indicated by laboratory values
- Therapeutic duplication
- Other contraindications

If any of these issues arise, it doesn't necessarily mean that the medication cannot be dispensed. However, your organization needs to develop a process to contact the prescriber in question and ensure that any issues are resolved. And you may want to document interventions taken if the medication is dispensed regardless of these issues.

See Figure 5-1 for a quick overview of the order review process.

Resolution of Issues

The review process may raise one or more concerns with the medication order, such as the following:

- The medication order is incomplete or unclear.
- The ordered medication has the same intended effect as another medication the patient is already taking.
- The ordered medication has a potentially harmful interaction with a medication the patient is already taking.
- The dosage or frequency ordered is concerning for a particular patient.

The pharmacist needs to resolve any questions or concerns that arise during the review process with the prescriber before the

The health care and human services fields are vast and provide care, treatment, and services to many individuals who may be referred to as patients, individuals served, residents, consumers, or clients. The term patient *is used throughout this book to describe a recipient of care, treatment, and services.*

?

Smart Questions

How does a pharmacist access patient information needed to perform order reviews?

in other words

therapeutic duplication
Prescribing more than one medication for the same indication or purpose.

picture this

Figure 5-1. Critical Questions in the Order Review Process

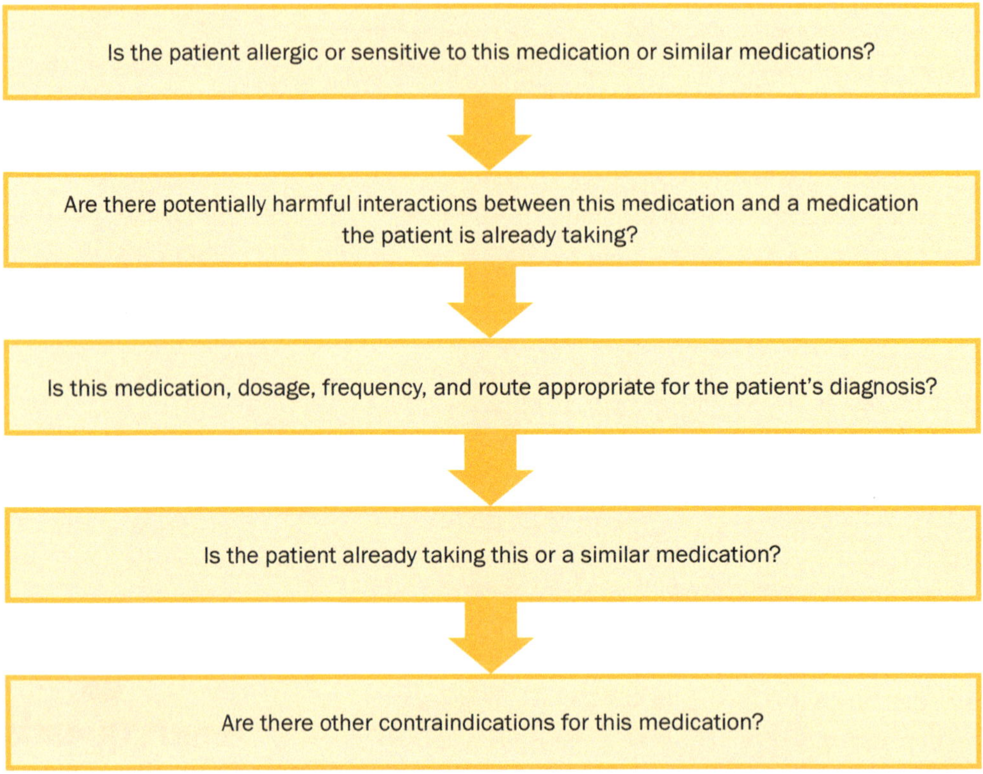

Smart Questions

What is the procedure for resolving issues raised during order reviews?

What are the procedures if you cannot immediately reach the prescriber?

medication is dispensed. And it's a good practice, although not required, to have a formal policy that addresses how these issues will be resolved and if documentation is required, including how the pharmacy will contact the prescriber and a time frame for resolving issues.

Exceptions

There are exceptions to the medication order review requirements addressed in the previous section. Here are just a couple of significant ones that apply to hospitals and critical access hospitals:

1. In some cases a licensed independent practitioner controls the ordering, preparation, and administration of a patient's medication. The practitioner may designate a qualified staff member, such as a registered nurse, to administer the medication. Although practitioners are not required to remain at the bedside when the medication is administered, they must be available to provide immediate intervention should a patient experience an adverse drug event.
2. In emergency situations, such as a sudden negative change in a patient's status, when a delay might harm the patient, staff may administer the medication without waiting for a full review.

Smart Questions

In what circumstances may your staff administer medications without pharmacist review?

Do you have a procedure for retroactively reviewing emergency or after-hours administrations of medication?

KEY CONCEPT

Safe Preparation of Medication Orders

Safe preparation of medications is critically important to patient safety. In all settings and situations, medications should be prepared and dispensed in the simplest, most ready-to-administer forms, such as pre-drawn syringes, individually packaged or dispensed capsules or tablets, and so on. When possible, you should discourage the admixture of medication components in areas outside the pharmacy, as this practice tends to increase variation and the probability of error. It may not be possible to eliminate all admixture outside the pharmacy, particularly in emergency departments or emergency situations. In such settings, staff members who work in departments or areas where these situations are likely to occur should be trained properly to perform the task.

In opioid treatment programs, licensed clinical staff other than a pharmacist (typically nursing staff) is permitted to prepare and dispense methadone, according to state and/or federal law and regulation.

Developing Safe Practices

In all areas where medications are prepared, staff should use aseptic techniques and maintain clean, uncluttered, and functionally separate workspaces to prevent contaminating each other's work during preparation. While staff members are preparing medications, they can inspect them for particulates, discoloration, or loss of integrity.

A 2020 survey by the Institute for Safe Medication Practices (ISMP) identified a number of common concerns related to safe and sterile preparation of medications.* These were concerns

* Institute for Safe Medication Practices. ISMP Survey Provides Insights into Preparation and Admixture Practices OUTSIDE the Pharmacy. Nov 4, 2020. Accessed Sep 23, 2021. https://www.ismp.org/resources/ismp-survey-provides-insights-preparation-and-admixture-practices-outside-pharmacy

picture this

Figure 5-2. Top Concerns of Survey Respondents for Medication Preparation

Area of Concern	Recommendations for Action
Lack of space	Ensure that staff inside and outside of the pharmacy, if applicable, have adequate space to prepare medications while minimizing the risk of contamination. Separate workspaces so that staff members are far enough away from one another and other possible sources of contaminants (for example, water).
Rushing through the preparation process	In the pharmacy, make sure you have adequate staff to handle the anticipated workload. Identify times when volume is likely to be high, and staff the pharmacy accordingly. Outside the pharmacy, make sure that staff members who may need to prepare medications in an emergency are trained properly to do so, and develop procedures and tools (for example, instructions, checklists, and so on) to help them complete the process quickly and accurately.
Mixing by memory	Develop written procedures for mixing medication preparations, and provide staff with tools to help them adhere to the procedures.
Interruptions or distractions	The design of workspaces in the pharmacy should take into account the need for a high degree of concentration. Such measures as limiting traffic in and out of preparation zones can help reduce distractions.
Incorrect preparation	Preparing only one medication at a time can help reduce the risk of preparation errors, such as getting the concentration wrong or using an incorrect diluent or other component.

Source: Adapted from Institute for Safe Medication Practices. ISMP Survey Provides Insights into Preparation and Admixture Practices OUTSIDE the Pharmacy. Nov 4, 2020. Accessed Sep 23, 2021. https://www.ismp.org/resources/ismp-survey-provides-insights-preparation-and-admixture-practices-outside-pharmacy.

raised about the preparation of medications outside the pharmacy, but they could apply within the pharmacy as well. To help you develop safe medication preparation practices, Figure 5-2 lists some of the prominent concerns raised by ISMP survey respondents and recommendations for addressing them.

KEY CONCEPT

Labeling Medications

Clear and complete medication labeling is foundational to medication safety. Every medication container must have a label that identifies the contents and provides other relevant information. Your medication management team can work together to decide what your labeling standard will be and what information you will require for a label to be considered complete. Joint Commission Medication Management (MM) standards have labeling requirements that are detailed in the sections that follow.

Minimum Requirements

Unless an authorized staff member is going to prepare or obtain a medication, take it directly to a patient, and administer it, without any break in the process, dispensed medications require a label. The information on that label must be in a standardized format. You can work with your medication management team to decide what format works best for your organization or setting. However, you should familiarize yourself with any applicable laws, regulations, and industry best practices for labeling and let that knowledge, as well as the experience and expertise of staff, inform your decisions.

Joint Commission Standard MM.05.01.09, Element of Performance (EP) 3,* indicates that a proper medication label must contain the following:

- Medication name
- Medication strength
- Medication amount (if not clear from the container)
- Expiration date when not used within 24 hours
- Expiration date and time when expiration occurs within 24 hours
- Date prepared
- Diluent for all compounded intravenous admixtures and parenteral nutrition formulas

If you're preparing individualized medications for multiple patients, or the person preparing the medication is different from the one who will administer it, the label should include these elements as well (in accordance with MM.05.01.09, EP 7):

- Patient name
- Location where the medication is to be delivered (for inpatient settings)

---

* This is not a requirement for assisted living communities.

- Directions for use
- Applicable accessory instructions
- Cautionary instructions

According to National Patient Safety Goal (NPSG) Standard NPSG.03.04.01, EP 3,* additional requirements for medication labels in perioperative and other procedural settings include the following:

- Medication or solution name
- Strength
- Amount of medication or solution containing medication (if not apparent from container)
- Diluent name and volume (if not apparent from container)
- Expiration date when not used within 24 hours
- Expiration time when expiration occurs in less than 24 hours

Review and Continuous Improvement

By monitoring how medications move through your medication management system and collecting data on risk, error, and patient harm, you can work to improve your labeling protocols. For example, maybe your labels need more information. Perhaps they need less, for clarity's sake. Or maybe the layout of label information needs to be adjusted, such as using special character sets to avoid look-alike/sound-alike confusion (see Chapter 4, page 57, for more information on look-alike/sound-alike medications).

Establish a periodic review of your labeling guidelines to make sure they are working as they should. Gather input from all the stakeholders, and work to improve this system on a regular basis.

Smart Questions

How does your organization make decisions about what information to include on medication labels?

Who makes these decisions?

KEY CONCEPT

Dispensing Medications

Safe, accurate, and timely dispensing of medications is a primary function of the pharmacy. Medications should be dispensed only in the quantities necessary to meet the needs of your patients. You need to keep clear and accurate records of all medications you dispense, in accordance with law, regulation, professional standards of practice, and organization policy.

Again, every organization and setting is different. For instance, home care organizations or behavioral health care and human

* This is not a requirement for assisted living communities, behavioral health care and human services organizations, home care organizations, or nursing care centers.

services facilities may not operate their own pharmacies. They need to define a process for obtaining needed medications in a timely way, whenever patients may need them.

You also must monitor performance to see whether the pharmacy is meeting expectations related to safe, accurate, and timely dispensing of medications. If not, you should explore why. Perhaps the time frame is unreasonable, given the requirements of safe preparation. Or maybe certain medication orders are coming in when the pharmacy is closed, and you don't have a solid process for handling these situations. Whatever the case, monitoring, documenting, and improving performance are important activities to ensure that patients are getting their medications when they are needed.

Finally, you want to consider the needs of the person administering the medication—whether that is a staff member, the patient, or a caregiver. Make sure the medication is dispensed in the most easily administrable form available, and, whenever you can, in unit doses. This provides a further check to ensure accurate dosing.

Multidose Vials

In some cases, you may want to dispense injectable medications in multidose vials (MDVs). In some settings, Joint Commission standards require that MDVs are used within 28 days, unless specified by the manufacturer. In settings that do not have specific Joint Commission requirements related to MDVs, you will need to follow manufacturers' instructions on preparation and administration. The Centers for Disease Control and Prevention (CDC) also has a number of recommendations for using MDVs, including the following:*

- A new sterile needle and syringe must be used for each administration.
- When the container is punctured, an updated expiration date must be determined and applied to the container.
- Vials must be discarded after 28 days, unless the manufacturer specifies a longer or shorter time period.
- If there is any question about the sterility of the medication, the vial should be discarded, regardless of date.

---

* Centers for Disease Control and Prevention. Injection Safety: Questions About Multi-Dose Vials. Jun 20, 2019. Accessed Sep 23, 2021. https://www.cdc.gov/injectionsafety/providers/provider_faqs_multivials.html.

MDVs in patient care areas should be dedicated to a single patient whenever possible. If you must use MDVs for more than one patient, they should not be kept in the immediate treatment area. This will help prevent accidental contamination of the vial through direct or indirect contact with potentially contaminated surfaces or equipment that could then lead to infection in other patients.

If an MDV enters the immediate treatment area of a patient, it must be dedicated to that individual only and discarded after use. Examples of immediate treatment areas include patient rooms or bays and operating rooms. When a medication is accessed in a direct care area, the vials are considered single use and are discarded on completion of that patient's case.

For more on this topic, visit the CDC Injection Safety webpage at https://www.cdc.gov/injectionsafety/ip07_standardprecaution.html.

in other **words**

automatic dispensing cabinet
Computerized medication storage devices or cabinets that allow medications to be stored or dispensed near the point of care, while controlling and tracking medication distribution. Also known as automated dispensing cabinet.

multidose vial
A vial of liquid medication intended for injection or infusion that contains more than one dose of medication.

TRY THIS TOOL

Tool 5-1. Automatic Dispensing Cabinets Override Review Policy

This sample policy provides a place to start when developing an ADC override policy for your organization. Be sure to adapt it to suit the needs and requirements of your organization.

Automatic Dispensing Cabinets

Many organizations have turned to automatic dispensing cabinets (ADCs) to streamline dispensing and to reduce error rates. In general, orders for medications dispensed through ADCs should still be reviewed by a pharmacist. However, in some situations, such as medical emergencies, you may need a certain medication very quickly. To deal with this in a safe way, your organization should create a list of acceptable medications and situations for which an override of the normal review process is acceptable. As part of your performance improvement process, you'll need to review these overrides periodically for appropriateness. You don't need to review every override. However, according to MM.08.01.01, EP 16,* you do need a written policy detailing what kinds of overrides you will review and how often.

ADCs have been instrumental in reducing variation in the dispensing process. But they should still be subject to the normal medication management system performance reviews to ensure that they and the protocols surrounding their use are serving the purposes set forth by the organization.

* This is not a requirement for office-based surgery practices.

KEY CONCEPT

Obtaining Medications

In hospitals or other organizations that operate a 24-hour pharmacy, when a medication order is submitted, and any issues have been resolved, the medication will be dispensed by the pharmacy and delivered to the appropriate staff member according to organization policy. Some patient care areas also may have floor stock of certain high-demand medications. And some medications may be kept in ADCs, where authorized staff can obtain them as needed.

Depending on the nature of your work, the size of your organization, and other factors, you may not operate a pharmacy 24 hours a day, 7 days a week. But medication orders will continue to come in. A rural hospital emergency department may need medications while the pharmacy is closed. Individuals at a behavioral health care and human services facility may need ready access to medications for symptom control. How will you obtain medications in these situations? The best approach is to devise and implement a policy covering these and other instances to maintain safety and consistency.

According to Joint Commission Standard MM.05.01.13, EP 2 , when staff members or licensed independent practitioners who are not pharmacists are allowed to obtain medications while the pharmacy is closed, they must observe the following safeguards to maintain security and quality and reduce the potential for variation:

- Maintain a list of medications that are approved for after-hours availability.
- Store (and secure) approved medications outside the pharmacy to maintain the security of the pharmacy.
- Give access to these medications only to designated prescribers and nurses.
- Institute a second check by another individual, or use a secondary verification procedure such as bar coding, to reduce medication retrieval errors.
- Designate a qualified pharmacist to be on call to answer questions or provide medications not preapproved for after-hours retrieval, during hours when the pharmacy is closed. This individual may be at another location.

Your organization may be able to enforce some of these safeguards using features of the software that controls ADCs.

TRY THIS TOOL

Tool 5-2. After-Hours Dispensing Policy Development Checklist

This checklist can help get you started thinking about a policy that governs how staff will access necessary medications when the pharmacy is closed.

Tool 5-3. Mock Tracer Worksheet: Medication Dispensing

Use this worksheet to help you assess your medication dispensing performance and identify areas for improvement.

Smart Questions

What medications are approved for after-hours orders?

What is the approval process?

Although the implementation of digital pharmacy information and ordering systems can help reduce variation in the ordering and transcribing process, no system is perfect. And when the order is received, it takes the careful work of dedicated pharmacy professionals, adhering to solid policies, law and regulation, and industry best practices, to safely and accurately prepare, label, and dispense medications. The ability to do this with a high degree of accuracy and deliver these medications in a timely fashion are the hallmarks of good medication management.

Additional Resources

The US Food and Drug Administration (FDA) has extensive resources for the labeling of medication packaging and the dispensing of medication. https://www.fda.gov/drugs/laws-acts-and-rules/prescription-drug-labeling-resources

CHAPTER 6

Administering Medications

The primary goal of medication management is to safely administer the correct medication to the correct patient in the correct dosage at the correct time and via the correct route. In this chapter we explore Joint Commission standards and best practices for ensuring consistency and reducing variation—and thus potential for error—in the administration of medications. We look at documentation and reconciliation requirements, requirements for self-administered medications, and the special concerns for investigational medications.

KEY CONCEPTS

- Medication Administration Basics
- Administration Verification Process
- Medication Reconciliation
- Self-Administration and Medications from Home
- Investigational Medications

The Standards

Following are the relevant standards for the content in this chapter from your setting's *Comprehensive Accreditation Manual* or its E-dition® counterpart.

Standard	AHC	ALC	BHC	CAH	HAP	NCC	OBS	OME
MM.03.01.05 The [organization] safely controls medications brought into the hospital by patients, their families, or [licensed independent practitioners].	X	X	X	X	X	X	X	X
MM.06.01.01 The [organization] safely administers medications.	X	X	X	X	X	X	X	X
MM.06.01.03 Self-administered medications are administered safely and accurately.		X	X	X	X	X		X
MM.06.01.05 The [organization] safely manages investigational medications.	X		X	X	X	X	X	X
NPSG.03.06.01 Maintain and communicate accurate patient medication information.	X	X	X	X	X	X	X	X
PC.02.03.01 The [organization] provides patient education and training based on each patient's needs and abilities.	X	X	X*	X	X	X	X	X

AHC, Ambulatory Health Care; ALC, Assisted Living Community; BHC, Behavioral Health Care and Human Services; CAH, Critical Access Hospital; HAP, Hospital; MM, Medication Management; NCC, Nursing Care Center; NPSG, National Patient Safety Goals; OBS, Office-Based Surgery Practice; OME, Home Care; PC, Provision of Care, Treatment, and Services.

* This requirement appears in Care, Treatment, and Services (CTS) Standard CTS.04.01.03 in the *Comprehensive Accreditation Manual for Behavioral Health Care and Human Services*.

KEY CONCEPT

Medication Administration Basics

Safe medication administration to patients requires attention to detail and a solidly defined policy. Figure 6-1 on page 80 details "The Nine Rights of Medication Administration." These are the basic elements of a reliable medication administration process. They include patient identification using more than one patient identifier. The Nine Rights also cover checking the medication order to ensure that the correct medication is being given in the correct dosage, at the correct time, by the correct route. Staff should also verify the reason the medication is being given to make sure it matches up with the patient's diagnosis and status.

The health care and human services fields are vast and provide care, treatment, and services to many individuals who may be referred to as patients, individuals served, residents, consumers, or clients. The term patient *is used throughout this book to describe a recipient of care, treatment, and services.*

The Nine Rights are an expanded version of the original Five Rights—which is what Joint Commission Medication Management (MM) Standard MM.06.01.01 is based on. Some organizations have gone beyond the Nine Rights to include other rights, such as the right to refuse medication.

Proper documentation of this whole process, including the preadministration process, patient vital signs, and other relevant information, is essential in informing continuing care decisions. Robust patient education helps patients make informed decisions and engages them as part of their own care team. And a plan to monitor the patient's response to the medication that takes into account the patient's perceptions of effects and side effects, as well as information from the medical record, is required for hospitals by Joint Commission Provision of Care, Treatment, and Services (PC) Standard PC.01.02.01, Element of Performance (EP) 1.

Defining Staff Roles

One of the first steps toward maintaining consistency during medication administration is to identify which staff members can administer medications to patients and make sure they are properly trained and competent to do so. Joint Commission Standard MM.06.01.01, EP 1, requires organizations to define in writing who may administer medications. Furthermore, you need to adhere to law, regulation, and organization requirements in determining which staff members are allowed to administer medication on their own and which require supervision.

As mentioned earlier, your organization may determine that some situations and settings allow for self-administration of medications. We examine the rules for self-administration later in this chapter (see page 87). For now, it's enough to know that you need to inform everyone involved in the administration of medications which category they are assigned to and the designated capabilities they possess.

Smart Questions

Which job roles are allowed to administer medications?

Are certain roles limited in the type of medications they can administer?

Are there certain medications that require special training or qualifications to administer?

The Joint Commission and the Centers for Medicare & Medicaid Services (CMS) have specific requirements for hospices providing inpatient care in their own facilities and electing to use Joint Commission accreditation for CMS deemed status. In this case, the hospice must limit the list of authorized people to licensed nurses, licensed physicians, health care professionals in accordance with their scope of practice and state law, employees who have completed a state-approved training program in medication administration, or the patient.

Optimizing Smart Infusion Pump Safety with Dose Error Reduction Software

Many health care organizations have turned to "smart" infusion pumps to help reduce variation and error in the administration of intravenous medications. These pumps use information such as patient information, medication dosing guidelines, and organizational parameters to reduce errors in dosing and infusion rates. The software can also be programmed to automatically require pharmacist or physician review before beginning an infusion.

Technology alone cannot ensure patient safety, however. "Smart" infusion pumps generally include dose error reduction software (DERS), which can identify human programming errors, yet substantial error rates persist because organizations are not optimizing the use of DERS. Of particular concern is the bypassing of "smart" pumps or the drug libraries programmed into them, which contain dosage and other safety information about individual medications. These libraries are intended to eliminate dosing and other administration errors by automating and/ or restricting some aspects of the administration process.

(continued)

picture this

Figure 6-1. The Nine Rights of Medication Administration

1. **Right Patient:** Check the identity of the patient and the medication order.
2. **Right Medication:** Check the medication order and label, as well as patient's allergies, before preparing medication.
3. **Right Dose:** Check the medication order, and calculate the dose. Double-check the dose when possible and always with high-alert medications.
4. **Right Time:** Check the medication order for instructions on optimal timing of the medication.
5. **Right Route:** Check the medication order for information on medication form and route.
6. **Right Reason:** Check the rationale of the medication and the patient's history and need for the medication.
7. **Right Documentation:** Document the medication administered (or response with PRN orders), as well as relevant information such as vital signs and patient education.
8. **Right Patient Education:** Provide medication education based on the patient's needs, and check the patient's understanding of such information.
9. **Right Response:** Check medication's therapeutic effects and potential side and adverse effects and interactions. Plan the relevant monitoring of these effects.

Source: Adapted from Nordic Medication Educators Collaboration, 2015.

The Nine Rights of Medication Administration is a further development of the long-standing Five Rights of Medication Administration often used by nurses to govern their medication verification and administration procedures. The original Five Rights are in blue.

Optimizing Smart Infusion Pump Safety with Dose Error Reduction Software (continued)

The Joint Commission has issued a *Sentinel Event Alert* (https://www.jointcommission.org/resources/patient-safety-topics/sentinel-event/sentinel-event-alert-newsletters/sentinel-event-alert-63-optimizing-smart-infusion-pump-safety-with-ders/) covering the optimization of DERS when using "smart" infusion pumps. If your organization makes use of "smart" infusion pumps and DERS, refer to the recommendations on the *Alert* to help reduce misuse and error.

in other **words**

informed consent

Agreement by patients to undergo a specific treatment or participate in an investigation, after they have been thoroughly educated as to its potential risk and benefits

KEY CONCEPT

Administration Verification Process

Before a medication is given to a patient, the nurse or other care provider must ensure that the medication being given conforms to the medication order. This review includes checking the following elements on the medication against the medication order:

- Medication
- Dosage
- Route of administration
- Time and frequency of administration
- Identity of the patient

The individual administering the medication should inform the patient about the medication and give the patient an opportunity to ask any questions.

Smart Questions

How will those tasked with administration of medications verify that they have the correct patient?

What is your organization's preadministration verification process?

How do you assess staff compliance with preadministration procedures?

At this point the nurse or other provider should assess the medication related to its appropriateness for the patient. Joint Commission Standard MM.06.01.01, EP 3, requires that the individual administering the medication do the following before giving the medication to the patient:

- Verify that the medication selected matches the medication order and product label.
- Visually inspect the medication for particulates, discoloration, or other loss of integrity.
- Verify that the medication has not expired.

- Verify that no contraindications exist.
- Verify that the medication is being administered at the proper time, in the prescribed dose, and by the correct route.
- Discuss any unresolved concerns about the medication with the patient's licensed independent practitioner, prescriber (if different), and/or staff involved with the patient's care, treatment, and services.

Documentation after you administer the medication is part of the process too. This complete process is shown in Figure 6-2 below.

TRY THIS TOOL

Tool 6-1. Preadministration Checklist

Use this checklist to review the necessary criteria you need to meet prior to administering medication.

picture this

Figure 6-2. Medication Administration Verification Process

BEFORE
Administering Medications

Verify that the medication **matches** the order for all its **elements:**
- Medication
- Dosage
- Route of administration
- Time and frequency of administration
- Identity of the patient

Inform the **patient** about the medication.

Give the **patient** the opportunity to ask **questions** about the medication.

AFTER
Administering Medications

Document the administered dose in the patient's **record** or on a **medication form**.

If your organization uses a separate **medication form**, add the form to the patient's **record** when the patient is **discharged** or **transferred**.

TRY THIS TOOL

Tool 6-2. Mock Tracer Worksheet: Medication Administration

This mock tracer worksheet is intended to help you assess the quality and performance of your medication administration system. Feel free to adapt it for your own use.

in other **words**

continuum of care

A concept that describes the movement of a patient through all phases and levels of health care, which seeks to join all the phases, levels, and organizations into an integrated whole for the purpose of the patient's care, treatment, or services.

medication reconciliation

The process of creating the most accurate list possible of all medications a patient is taking—including medication name, dosage, frequency, and route—and comparing that list against the admission, transfer, and/or discharge orders, with the goal of providing correct medications to the patient at all transition points within the organization.

Also, if the medication is a new one for the patient, a staff member needs to have a conversation with the patient or the patient's family or guardian about possible significant adverse drug reactions and any other concerns raised by the new medication. This helps patients make informed decisions about their care, treatment, or services.

KEY CONCEPT

Medication Reconciliation

As patients move through the continuum of care, managing their medications can be challenging (see Figure 6.3 on page 85 for examples of possible problems and errors). Medication reconciliation involves creating an accurate list of all medications a patient is taking prior to admission or the start of an encounter, including name, dosage, frequency, and route, and comparing that list against the physician's admission or discharge orders in the patient's medical record. Medication information should also be reconciled at patient discharge or the end of an encounter. (The specific requirements for reconciliation can be found in Joint Commission National Patient Safety Goal 3 [NPSG.03.06.01].)

There are often a lot of people involved in the care of a single patient in a single episode of care or over multiple episodes of care, and these people need to accurately communicate critical information about which medications the patient is taking to avoid problems such as improper dosing, timing errors, or harmful drug interactions. Medication reconciliation aims to reduce the potential for error that is associated with a patient's transition of care.

Staff Roles in Medication Reconciliation

The process of compiling a list of the medications a patient is taking—which is then reviewed to determine future prescribing decisions—is a point of significant risk of error. Information from patients and caregivers may be incomplete or incorrect, and when medication orders are transcribed, errors can occur, such as missing decimal points or incorrect route for administration. Therefore, this is a part of the process that deserves special attention.

If possible, it's a good idea to establish the process of compiling and communicating this medication list as a specific role for certain staff members to resolve any questions, concerns, or discrepancies. Likewise, it's helpful to involve a pharmacist in this process. Pharmacists' training and experience can help them spot possible errors in dosages or routes, potential drug interactions, and other issues that may not be immediately apparent to others.

Thorough Medication Documentation

In addition to the names, dosages, routes, and frequencies of each medication, it is important to include the purpose of each medication in the patient's medication list as part of the reconciliation process. Patients may have multiple diagnoses and may be taking an array of medications to treat them. Part of the purpose of medication reconciliation is to determine not just what medications the patient is taking but also what medications are

picture this

Figure 6-3. Potential Medication Reconciliation Problems and Errors

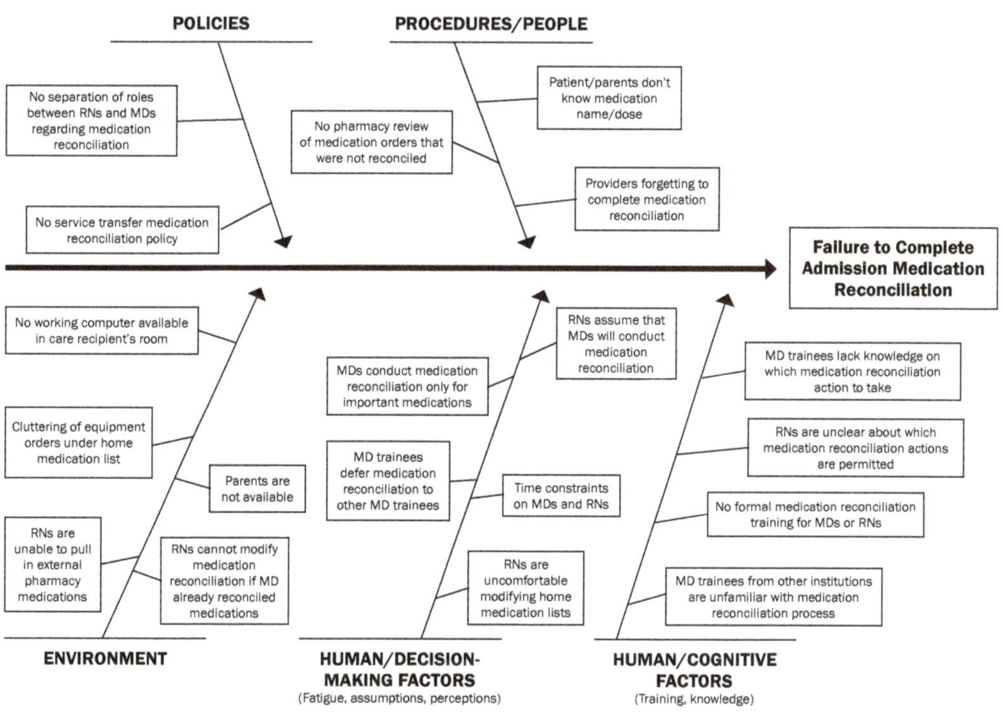

This fishbone diagram illustrates several important factors that can contribute to medication reconciliation problems and errors.

picture this

Figure 6-4. Medication Reconciliation Process

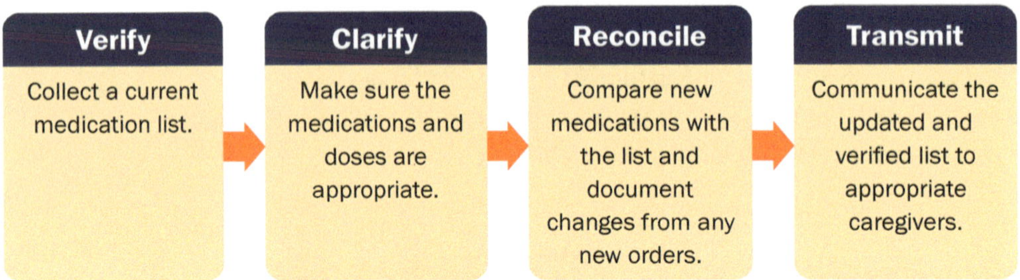

This figure shows the essential elements of medication reconciliation.

appropriate, what medications may be stopped, and what medications should be started or substituted. Medication reconciliation is meant to help ensure that no medications are omitted from the patient's plan of care. Matching up the patient's medications with his or her diagnoses, and including this information in the patient's plan of care, helps reduce errors and omissions—as well as duplications—and helps the care team think about the purpose and goals of treatment.

Smart Questions

What process do you use for medication reconciliation?

Who is responsible for collecting the information about what the patient takes at home, for reconciling this with new prescriptions that will be written, and for creating a home medication list at the end of the encounter?

Where is the medication reconciliation documented?

How do you communicate information about a change in a patient's medication regimen at admission, discharge, or visit?

Medication Education

Patients and their families are an integral part of the medication reconciliation process. When medications are prescribed by your organization, you need to give medication information to patients and/or their families at discharge. Standard PC.02.03.01, EP 10, requires certain organizations to provide information and education on the safe and effective use of medications. For behavioral health care and human services organizations, Care, Treatment, and Services (CTS) Standard CTS.04.01.03, EP 4, requires patient education, including medication education, where appropriate. In addition, NPSG.03.06.01 requires you to provide the following:

- Written information about the medications the patient or individual should be taking
- Education about how to manage the patient's medication information (such as maintaining a current list of medications)

KEY CONCEPT

Self-Administration and Medications from Home

Self-Administration

Self-administration is another area in which education is critical to maintaining patient safety. According to MM.06.01.03, EP 3,* before you authorize patients and/or their families to self-administer, you need to provide them with information on the following:

- The types, names, and reasons for use of any medications given
- How to administer the medication safely, including the process for how to administer it, the time, the frequency, the route, and the dose
- What to expect after the medication is administered, including any common side effects
- How to monitor themselves (or their family member) after administration, including knowing how side effects manifest and how to tell if the medication is working
- How to document the administration

You will also need to develop supports and materials to help deliver this patient information to patients with limited English proficiency, including interpretation services, where available and appropriate.

It's a good idea to have some form of formal competency assessment that must be met before self-administration can occur. You should also develop a written policy to help ensure safe administration of these medications. The policy should include criteria for determining who is eligible to self-administer, what training you will provide to patients and/or family members before authorizing them to administer, and specific staff responsibilities for recording information about medications brought from home and monitoring patients. For more information about developing a self-administration policy, see Tool 6-3 on page 88.

in other **words**

self-administration

Independent use of a medication by a patient, resident, or individual served, including medications that may be held by the organization for independent use.

* This is not a requirement for ambulatory health care centers or office-based surgery practices.

TRY THIS TOOL

Tool 6-3. Self-Administered Medications Policy

Use this sample tool as you develop a policy on the self-administration of medications. Be sure to adapt it to suit the needs and requirements of your organization and local laws and regulations.

Smart Questions

What documentation do you require to show that patients have received the necessary education to enable them to self-administer medications?

How do you assess patients' competency related to self-administering medications?

What provisions have you made to ensure that patient education is available to individuals with limited English proficiency?

Do you offer interpretation services or patient educational materials in languages other than English that are prevalent in your area?

Self-Administration in Behavioral Health Care and Human Services Organizations

Behavioral health care and human services organizations commonly employ some version of self-administration, whether individuals are managing, storing, and dispensing their medications fully on their own, or staff is storing and dispensing medications for them to administer themselves. Self-administration in these settings depends on a number of factors, including organization policy, services provided, population served, and so on.

Managing the Risks of Oral Anticoagulants

The use of direct oral anticoagulants (DOACs) to treat a variety of conditions has been rising in recent years. The convenience of prescribing medications that patients can administer to themselves has been a driving factor in the expansion of their use. However, as the use of DOACs has increased, so has the occurrence of adverse drug events related to them.

The danger often arises when a patient has a bleeding event, such as intracranial bleeding associated with head trauma. Although a variety of DOACs have come into common use in recent years, clinicians are not always aware of the specific characteristics, indications for use, and reversal strategies of these medications. The reversal strategies of DOACs may be substantially different from one another and, importantly, from warfarin or heparin, anticoagulants clinicians may be more familiar with.

The Joint Commission has issued a *Sentinel Event Alert* (https://www.jointcommission.org/resources/patient-safety-topics/sentinel-event/sentinel-event-alert-newsletters/sentinel-event-alert-61-managing-the-risks-of-direct-oral-anticoagulants/) covering the use of DOACs, which contains guidance on how to design protocols for the use of DOACs. Refer to the *Alert* for recommended protocols and enhanced patient education recommendations.

Because indications for use and reversal strategies for DOACs may differ substantially from other anticoagulants and each other, extra care and solid policy are needed to prevent avoidable errors when using these therapies.

Medications from Home

Patients bring their own medications from home for a variety of reasons. One reason is to show their provider which medications they are currently taking (this helps create the home medication list described on page 84). Other patients wish to take a medication that is not available in your organization.

Your organization should have a process for dealing with medication patients or caregivers bring from home. At a minimum, according to MM.03.01.05, the organization must define when medications brought into the organization can be administered. This includes evaluating whether each medication should be taken and documenting the reasons why or why not. In addition, each medication brought in should be visually inspected by staff for particulates, contamination, loss of integrity, and so on. Then staff should determine when, how, and by whom any medications brought in by patients or caregivers will be administered.

If medications brought from home are approved for self-administration, all of the precautions outlined in the section on self-administration should be observed, including patient education and a self-administration competency assessment (see page 87).

KEY CONCEPT

Investigational Medications

Investigational medications are drugs that are approved by the US Food and Drug Administration (FDA) for use as part of a research protocol or clinical trial. In some situations, a patient may be enrolled in a clinical trial that involves the use of an investigational medication, or a provider might prescribe an investigational medication on a compassionate basis. Of course, any time you're administering a new medication to a patient, there is some element of increased risk. And with investigational medications, you need to take extra steps to ensure that administration is done safely and the rights of your patient are respected by authorized staff.

In the case of clinical trials, the trial itself must be reviewed and overseen by an Institutional Review Board (IRB), and a patient education and consent process for each patient in the trial must be approved by the IRB.

in other **words**

investigational medication
A medication used as part of a research protocol or clinical trial.

TRY THIS TOOL

Tool 6-4. Investigational Medications Process Checklist

Use this checklist to ask key questions when developing a written process for using investigational medications. Be sure to understand your organization's legal obligations when it comes to clinical trials.

Investigational medications may be a good option for patients with few other options. Issues of ethics, informed consent, and patient's rights must be addressed to make sure that the patient, the care team, and the organization are on the same page when choosing this option. Care providers need to make sure that patients understand the possible risks and benefits of investigational medications, possible side effects, available alternative courses of treatment, and their rights if they do choose to participate in a trial, including their right to opt out of the trial after it has begun without penalty or other adverse effect on their care and treatment. If your organization decides to make investigational medications available to your patients, Joint Commission Standard MM.06.01.05 requires a written process to govern their use.

Smart Questions

Do you have a standing body to consider which investigations or studies your organization will participate in?

How is that body constituted?

Clinical Trials

The process for the design, review, approval, and oversight of clinical trials is strictly governed by federal law. You'll need to familiarize yourself with applicable law if your organization will be running or participating in clinical trials. In addition, your written process on investigational medications must state that the pharmacy controls the storage, dispensing, labeling, and distribution of investigational medications. As in other areas of medication management, controlling who has access to the medication, how it is dispensed, and when it is administered is a key part of keeping variation low and maintaining patient safety. And, in the case of clinical trials, it helps ensure the integrity of the study.

Finally, your written process should spell out the relationship between patients, the organization, and those running the study. When patients are involved in a clinical trial or investigational study that is not being run by your organization, appropriate staff members evaluate patients' continued participation in the protocol. Barring any contraindication, they allow patients to continue in the protocol. When patients are enrolled in the study, they stay in the study unless there is a reason to pull them out. These decisions may not be easy or clear and, therefore, should be plainly defined in your written process.

Smart Questions

What procedures do you have in place to ensure that patients' rights are protected and their informed consent is obtained when they are considering participating in an investigational study?

The administration of medications is among the highest-risk activities that regularly fall among the duties of an organization's staff. With a solid policy and procedures in place that incorporate the patient's medication management rights and adheres to law, regulation, and Joint Commission standards, many medication

Sample Medications

Some organizations receive samples of medications from manufacturers or vendors. Prescribers can choose to dispense or administer these sample medications to their patients. Because such medications may be new to the organization, special care should be taken in the storage, handling, and use of sample medications. Your organization should consider whether it will allow the use of sample medications, and if so, develop policies and procedures to guide the approved use of medication samples within the organization.

There are notes in the MM standards of your *Comprehensive Accreditation Manual* showing which standards and EPs apply to sample medications. Special areas concerning the administration of sample medications include the following:

- The heightened risk of harmful drug interactions when using a medication new to the market, prescriber, or organization
- Clarity of instructions for use, particularly as many sample medications will be prescribed for self-administration
- Patient education in the administration of sample medications and monitoring for effects
- The inclusion of sample medications in medication lists used for reconciliation

errors can be prevented. With proper monitoring, the effects of medication errors or adverse events that do occur can be substantially mitigated. And regular medication reconciliation can help reduce adverse events and keep the patient and care team focused on the patient's care goals. Robust policies covering self-administration and investigation medications are also critical to patient safety.

Additional Resources

Joint Commission *Sentinel Event Alert* 63 addresses the optimization of dose error reduction software (DERS) when using "smart" infusion pumps. https://www.jointcommission.org/resources/patient-safety-topics/sentinel-event/sentinel-event-alert-newsletters/sentinel-event-alert-63-optimizing-smart-infusion-pump-safety-with-ders/

CHAPTER 7

Monitoring Patients' Reactions

When an adverse drug event or medication error occurs, quickly responding to the event can be a critical factor in preventing or reducing harm to the patient. Therefore, it's essential that you establish a robust system of monitoring how patients react to their medications. The system should be set up to ensure that the following occurs in the event of an adverse drug reaction:

- Notify the appropriate people.
- Carry out mandatory reporting.
- Gather data to help your organization treat patients and improve monitoring systems.

In this chapter, we introduce you to some of the basic elements of patient monitoring and responses to adverse drug events.

KEY CONCEPTS

- Plan to Monitor Patient Response
- Adverse Drug Event Response

The Standards

Following are the relevant standards for the content in this chapter from your setting's *Comprehensive Accreditation Manual* or its E-dition® counterpart.

Standard	AHC	ALC	BHC	CAH	HAP	NCC	OBS	OME
MM.07.01.01 The [organization] monitors patients to determine the effects of their medication(s).	X		X	X		X	X	X
MM.07.01.03 The [organization] responds to actual or potential adverse drug events, significant adverse drug reactions, and medication errors.	X	X	X	X	X	X		X

AHC, Ambulatory Health Care; ALC, Assisted Living Community; BHC, Behavioral Health Care and Human Services; CAH, Critical Access Hospital; HAP, Hospital; MM, Medication Management; NCC, Nursing Care Center; OBS, Office-Based Surgery Practice; OME, Home Care.

The health care and human services fields are vast and provide care, treatment, and services to many individuals who may be referred to as patients, individuals served, residents, consumers, or clients. The term patient *is used throughout this book to describe a recipient of care, treatment, and services.*

KEY CONCEPT

Plan to Monitor Patient Response

Monitoring is an important means of assessing how well a patient's medication regimen is working and to watch for any adverse side effects, interactions, or events. In fact, Joint Commission Medication Management (MM) Standard MM.07.01.01* requires this monitoring process in certain settings. The information you obtained about side effects, interactions, and so on when determining whether to add a medication to your formulary can be used to inform your monitoring activities.

A good plan designates which staff members are primarily responsible for monitoring patients. Patient monitoring is a team effort (see Figure 7-1 on page 96). Obviously, that team includes nurses, physicians, and other frontline staff. But there are also roles to play for pharmacists, medical specialists, and, as discussed below, patients and their caregivers. A solid plan also identifies the assessments staff members will perform, clarifies the information they are seeking in such assessments, and provides criteria for measuring the effects and side effects of the medication.

* This is not a requirement for hospitals or assisted living communities.

Clarify how often and at what points during the continuum of care the monitoring activities should occur. Staff members will need support, such as forms or other tools, for recording data and observations; a way to access and compare previously collected data; and a method to convey this information to the attending physician, pharmacist, and other medication management team members.

It's a good idea to periodically review this monitoring plan to ensure that it's serving the needs of your organization and its processes are clear for those who are responsible for monitoring patients. Make sure these processes are in place before offering new medications on the medication formulary.

in other **words**

side effects

A secondary, typically undesirable effect of a medication or medical treatment.

Patient's Role in Monitoring

Some of the best sources of information about the effects and side effects of medications are patients—particularly if they have started a new medication. Monitoring a patient after the first dose of a medication is an important patient safety activity. During this assessment you may discover that the patient has a previously undetected sensitivity to the medication or that it has an unexpected and harmful interaction with a medication the patient is already taking. Whatever the case, asking patients questions about how they are feeling and their perceptions of how well the medication is working is a good way to obtain information about a medication's effects.

This kind of assessment should also be done periodically as part of the broader monitoring process. Also important are checking and documenting vital signs and other relevant values, as applicable to the care setting or service. These data, along with clinical observations, should be entered into the patient's medical record so they can be compared to earlier observations and measurements. Electronic monitoring systems can help with real-time monitoring of certain aspects of a patient's condition and alerting staff to sudden changes in condition.

Smart Questions

What extra monitoring measures do you require after the first dose of a new medication?

picture this

Figure 7-1. Interdisciplinary Monitoring Team

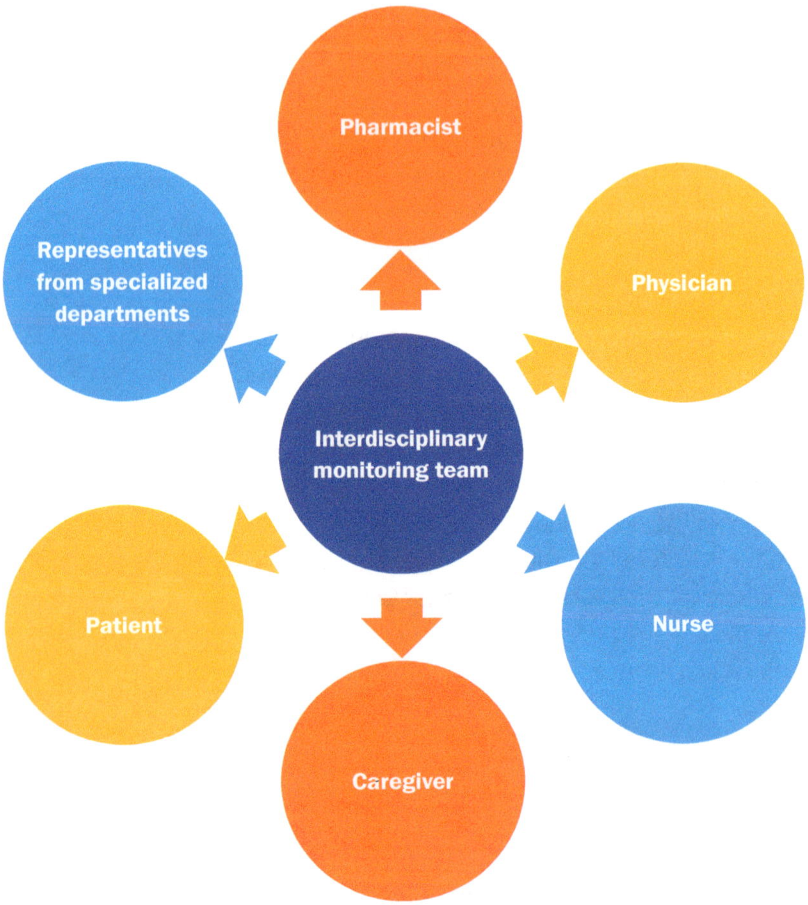

Good monitoring requires a team effort. It takes patients, caregivers, and nurses directly monitoring the patient. Pharmacists offer superior knowledge of medications and their effects and possible side effects. And physicians and members of specialty departments analyze monitoring information and decide when and how to react to changes in the patient's condition.

Long-Term Considerations

In some settings, such as nursing care centers, individuals may receive care over long periods of time, during which they receive different medications. Your patient monitoring plan should include a schedule for assessing a patient's entire medication regimen at least monthly. This is required by Joint Commission standards for nursing care centers (MM.07.01.01, Element of Performance [EP] 4), and it's a good idea in any setting where patients remain in care for long periods of time.

These long-term assessments should look at how well a medication regimen is serving the patient's health goals (see sidebar below), whether changes need to be made based on changes in the patient's condition or response to medications, and whether better alternatives exist to the medications currently being administered. This can be done as part of a broader periodic assessment of the patient's condition and/or specific responses to the progression of any conditions related to medications.

Age-Friendly Care and the 4Ms

As the number of adults over the age of 65 continues to rise rapidly in the United States, health care organizations and industry groups have been looking for ways to better serve older patients. One approach to age-friendly care, the 4Ms framework, was developed by a group of geriatrics experts and detailed in "Evidence for the 4Ms: Interactions and Outcomes Across the Care Continuum."* This approach to health care for older adults centers patient care around each individual patient's goals for quality of life and health care outcomes. The first of the 4Ms—What Matters—informs how you pursue the other three Ms: Medication, Mentation, and Mobility.

Medication is obviously a big part of the 4Ms approach. Decisions made by patients and their care team about medications profoundly affect Mobility, Mentation, and

* Mate K, et al. Evidence for the 4Ms: Interactions and outcomes across the care continuum. *J Aging Health*. 2021 Aug-Sep;33(7-8):469-481. Accessed Aug 18, 2021. https://doi.org/10.1177/0898264321991658.

Age-Friendly Care and the 4Ms (continued)

What Matters. Each time you have an interaction with a patient, you'll want to keep the 4Ms in mind and tailor any medication decisions to suit your patient's goals. This approach is a way of remembering that you are not treating a disease or condition but rather a person whose priorities may or may not include absolute control of every health care issue, particularly if that patient's medication regimen interferes with What Matters most to him or her.

For example, for some patients, you may want to avoid any medications that interfere with Mentation or Mobility, as these are critical to quality of life. Other patients may be willing to tolerate some limitations on Mobility for the security of knowing their condition is well controlled. Age-friendly care means talking to older patients, finding out what they want from their health care provider, and helping them get there.

TRY THIS TOOL

Tool 7-1. Sample Patient Monitoring Form

Use this sample form to record patient monitoring concerns and procedures.

KEY CONCEPT

Adverse Drug Event Response

Joint Commission Standard MM.07.01.03* requires organizations to devise and follow a written process to respond to actual or potential adverse drug events, significant adverse drug reactions, and medication errors. Depending on your patient population, the medications you regularly dispense, and other factors, your organization will have a specific risk profile for adverse drug reactions or events.

For instance, organizations that provide long term care for elderly residents may need to be extra vigilant about drug interactions because such residents tend to take more medications. Behavioral health care and human services organizations may place more emphasis on observing behavioral changes because they may be more likely to administer psychotropic medications. Home care staff might rely more on patient self-monitoring and reporting of side effects. And any organization where antibiotics

* This is not a requirement for office-based surgery practices.

are regularly prescribed needs to stay vigilant for adverse reactions caused by sensitivities, allergies, or other factors.

Reporting Medication Errors

In accordance with Standard MM.07.01.03, EP 3,* all staff members are required to report actual or potential adverse drug events, significant adverse drug reactions, and any medication errors. Keep in mind that staff and providers who are blamed for errors may be less inclined to report them. Lack of reporting such errors leads to more risk, particularly if the incidents actually have roots in system issues. Respecting those who report errors is part of a culture of safety.

For organizations that use Joint Commission accreditation for deemed status purposes, the Centers for Medicare & Medicaid Services (CMS) expects the attending physician or other provider to be immediately notified when harm to a patient has already occurred due to a medication error or where there is potential for harm as a result of the medication error. If the outcome of the error is unknown, the physician must still be notified immediately, as addressing the needs of the patient must be the priority.

When an adverse drug event happens, it is also important to notify the prescriber of the medication. Joint Commission Standard MM.07.01.03, EP 2,* requires organizations in certain settings to create and follow a written process that details how and when to notify the prescriber in the event of an adverse drug event, significant adverse drug reaction, or medication error. This is critical information for the prescriber to have when making further decisions about the patient's—or future patients'—medications and care. In the home care setting, the results of the monthly pharmacist's review of the patient's medication must also be communicated to the provider who is prescribing medications for that patient.

Understanding the Root Causes of Medication Errors

Knowing the most common causes of medication errors may help you focus on contributing factors within your organization. Awareness of the impact of blame in reporting errors can help to empower employees to report incidents without fear of retribution.

* This is not a requirement for office-based surgery practices.

in other words

adverse drug event
An injury resulting from a medical intervention related to a medication, including harm from an adverse drug reaction or a medication error.

adverse drug reaction
A response to a medicinal product that is noxious and unintended and that occurs at doses normally used in humans for the prophylaxis, diagnosis, or treatment of disease or for the restoration, correction, or modification of physiological or psychological function.

medication error
Any preventable event that may cause or lead to inappropriate medication use or patient harm while the medication is in the control of the health care professional or patient.

significant adverse drug reaction
A reaction in which the patient's outcome is death, life threatening, hospitalization, disability, congenital anomaly, or required intervention to prevent permanent impairment or damage.

Smart Questions

How do you notify prescribers following an adverse drug reaction?

Do your actions change depending on the severity of the reaction?

Smart Questions

Do incident reports provide meaningful data to use for improvement efforts?

How else might data be collected?

TRY THIS TOOL

Tool 7-2. Adverse Drug Event Processes Checklist

Use this sample checklist to develop standardized processes to respond to actual or potential adverse drug events and medication errors.

Tool 7-3. Medication Error Investigation Procedure Checklist

This checklist can be used to guide a multidisciplinary team when investigating how a medication error occurred. It does not take the place of an incident report form. Rather, it outlines the steps that could be used to meaningfully investigate an error to understand what happened, why, and how to prevent its recurrence. Ideally, the investigation should occur as soon as possible after the incident.

Tool 7-4. Medication Event Incident Report

Use this tool to document critical information related to an adverse drug event or other medication error.

Consider the following:

- **Provide education.** All providers, prescribers, and staff should be aware of when and how to report medication errors, according to your organization's policy. Provide in-service training on this topic frequently to make sure everyone is clear about what to do when mistakes occur.
- **Work with data.** Look at incident reports to see how errors are being categorized.

Obtain and document regular updates from patients and their families, as well as nursing and other staff, regarding medication side effects. In some settings, such as home care organizations or nursing care centers, Joint Commission standards require a pharmacist review of the patient's medications on at least a monthly basis. Pharmacist review is good practice in any setting and may need to be done more frequently in settings or cases when the patient's medication regimen changes more frequently, such as in opioid treatment programs, where a maintenance dose of medication may be determined by monitoring patient reaction. Physicians or other primary providers should regularly evaluate changes in the patient's status and use the patient's medical record to inform choices about changing the medication regimen.

Even with best practices in place that reduce variation and error, some patient harm related to medications may still occur. What actions will staff take to minimize harm to the patient? If it is not safe to stop a medication immediately, how will you mitigate patient harm? For safe, high-quality care, organizations must have processes in place to respond to and monitor a patient if an adverse reaction or event is underway.

Additional Resources

The Centers for Medicare & Medicaid Services Adverse Drug Event Trigger Tool can help identify patients who may have experienced an adverse drug reaction or adverse drug event and categorize the experience. The tool can also guide your thinking related to what level of severity might call for a response and what that initial response might look like. https://www.cms.gov/Medicare/Provider-Enrollment-and-Certification/QAPI/Downloads/Adverse-Drug-Event-Trigger-Tool.pdf

CHAPTER 8

Evaluating the Medication Management Process

As with any health care process, evaluation is essential to understanding how well you're doing. Because administering medications to patients involves, by its very nature, increased patient risk, pursuing continuous improvement in this area should be a major focus of performance improvement efforts across your organization. If you want to be a high reliability organization, you need to examine and analyze what you're doing, see what's working and what could be improved, and use that knowledge to reduce variation and risk, improve processes and policies, and foster a culture of safety.

KEY CONCEPTS

- Reporting Requirements
- Collecting Data
- Analyzing Data
- Identifying and Addressing Improvement Opportunities

The Standards

Following are the relevant standards for the content in this chapter from your setting's *Comprehensive Accreditation Manual* or its E-dition® counterpart.

Standard	AHC	ALC	BHC	CAH	HAP	NCC	OBS	OME
MM.08.01.01 The [organization] evaluates the effectiveness of its medication management system.	X	X	X	X	X	X	X	X

AHC, Ambulatory Health Care; ALC, Assisted Living Community; BHC, Behavioral Health Care and Human Services; CAH, Critical Access Hospital; HAP, Hospital; MM, Medication Management; NCC, Nursing Care Center; OBS, Office-Based Surgery Practice; OME, Home Care.

The health care and human services fields are vast and provide care, treatment, and services to many individuals who may be referred to as patients, individuals served, residents, consumers, or clients. The term patient *is used throughout this book to describe a recipient of care, treatment, and services.*

KEY CONCEPT

Reporting Requirements

Reporting adverse drug reactions and events and other medication errors to your medication management team and performance improvement team is an integral part of your patient safety and performance improvement activities. In fact, given the potential risk of patient harm that is associated with medication errors, the medication management system should be a special area of focus in your organization's performance improvement program. Depending on your state and health care setting, reporting such events may be required to comply with law and regulation (see Figure 8-1 on page 103 for a breakdown of required and voluntary reporting).

The *Survey Analysis for Evaluating Risk*® (*SAFER*®) Matrix that is provided by The Joint Commission after your organization's accreditation survey is one tool to use to identify risk. The *SAFER* Matrix provides one comprehensive visual representation of survey findings in which all Requirements for Improvement are plotted according to the likelihood of the issue to cause harm to patients, staff, or visitors, in addition to how widespread the problem is, based on surveyors' observations.

Being able to detect changes and trends in the rates of adverse events is key to identifying why these events are happening and how to reduce or eliminate them. Investigation techniques, such as root cause analysis, can help organizations gain a deeper understanding of how adverse events happen and how they can be prevented.

picture this

Figure 8-1. Reporting Options and Responsibilities

Required Reporting	Voluntary Reporting
• Leadership • Team responsible for medication management • Team tasked with performance improvement • Some state and federal government agencies	• The Joint Commission • Government agencies (for example, the US Food and Drug Administration) • Regional health care coalitions

Some adverse drug event (ADE) reporting is mandated by law or regulation, but your organization may choose to volunteer ADE data with a variety of entities. Sharing these data helps such organizations track trends in ADEs and develop guidance for organizations in reducing the frequency of such events.

Sentinel Event Reporting and Response

Sentinel event reporting is another kind of reporting to consider when evaluating your medication management process. The Joint Commission does not require organizations to report sentinel events as a condition for accreditation; it requires only that organizations internally respond to sentinel events, including medication-related events, with a comprehensive systematic analysis such as a root cause analysis (see Figure 8-2 on page 104 for the major steps in a root cause analysis and Tool 8-1 on page 104 for a root cause analysis checklist).

However, The Joint Commission collects sentinel event and other adverse event data so it can learn more about why sentinel events happen and how organizations can minimize their frequency and severity. The more data the sentinel event reporting program collects, the clearer the picture becomes and the more reliable the conclusions. The Joint Commission uses this information in its *Sentinel Event Alerts* to highlight areas of patient safety or patient risk that have come to The Joint Commission's attention, and it provides recommendations on how to avoid such areas.

?

Smart Questions

What are your criteria for reporting adverse drug events to your performance improvement team?

What improvement projects have you implemented to try to reduce adverse reactions and medication errors?

What is the process for reporting an adverse drug event or reaction to leadership? What is leadership's response?

In your locality, which state or federal reporting requirements apply?

picture this

Figure 8-2. Root Cause Analysis Process

Define the Event

What happened? Who was involved? Where did the event occur?

↓

Find Causes

What directly caused this event?

↓

Focus on Root Causes

What actions led to or contributed to this event?

↓

Find Solutions

How could this be prevented?

↓

Take Action

What are we going to do to avoid a similar event in the future?

↓

Verify Action Was Effective

Did the solution work?

Moving beyond blame after an adverse event is part of creating a safety culture. Root cause analysis is a tool for investigating why events occurred and identifying corrective actions. It is part of a process of accountability. This figure highlights the major steps in an effective root cause analysis.

TRY THIS TOOL

Tool 8-1. Medication Error Root Cause Analysis Checklist

Use this checklist to help start the discussion about the root causes of a medication error.

These *Alerts* contain information that is intended to help all organizations refine their systems and processes to prevent the worst and most common patient harm events. Figure 8-3 below shows the flow of the sentinel event reporting process.

picture this

Figure 8-3. The Joint Commission's Sentinel Event Process Flow

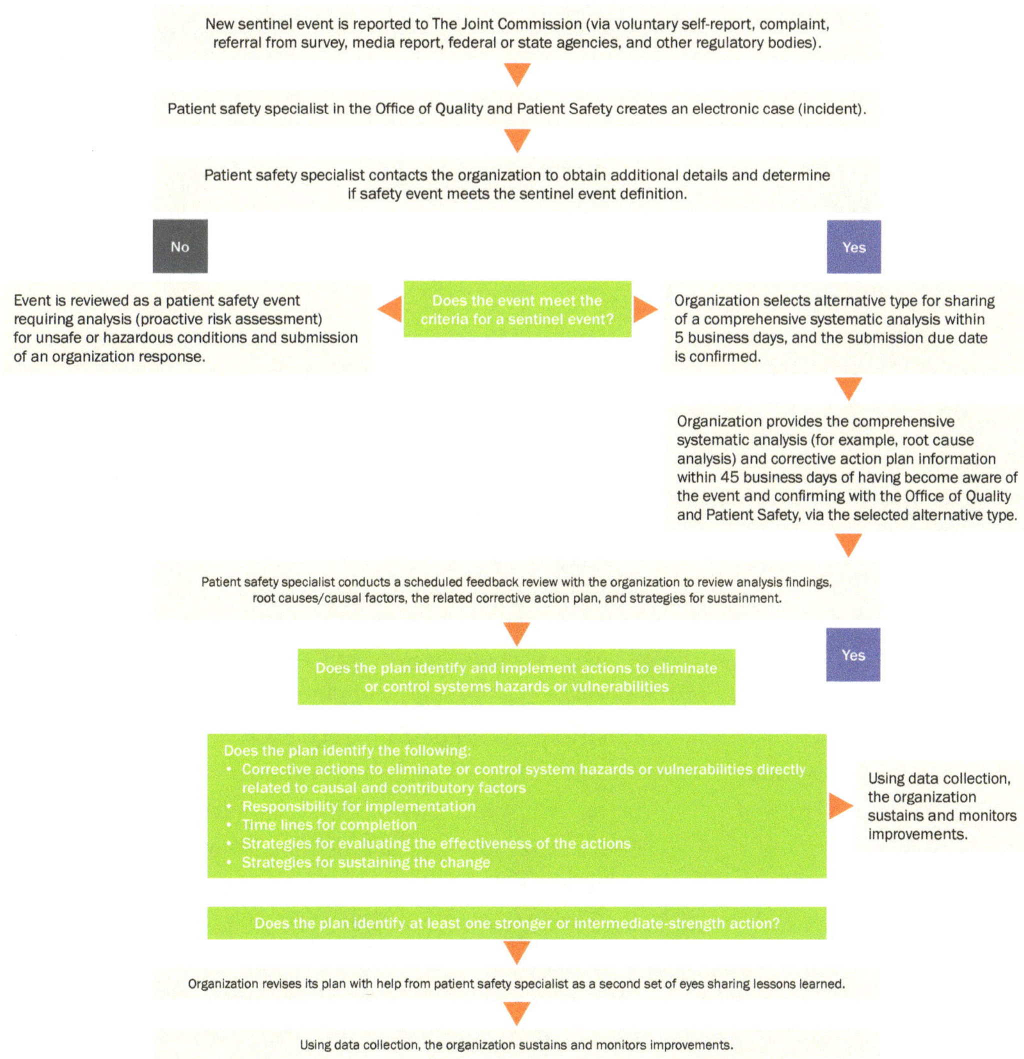

This flowchart gives a snapshot of the sentinel event reporting process to The Joint Commission.

in other words

root cause analysis
A process for identifying the basic or causal factors underlying variation in performance, including the occurrence or possible occurrence of a sentinel event.

sentinel event
A patient safety event (not primarily related to the natural course of the patient's illness or underlying condition) that reaches a patient and results in death, severe harm (regardless of duration of harm), or permanent harm (regardless of severity of harm).

Smart Questions

Which medication processes are you going to evaluate?

Which data need to be collected to evaluate the performance of those processes?

How can you make it easier to report, collect, and organize medication management data?

Which technology resources can you leverage to gather these data and transform them into information?

Please refer to the Sentinel Event Policy in the "Sentinel Event Policy" (SE) chapter of your *Comprehensive Accreditation Manual* or its E-dition counterpart for the most up-to-date criteria organizations use to develop root cause analyses and address vulnerabilities with corrective action plans.

KEY CONCEPT

Collecting Data

We can't overstate the importance of collecting data on the medication management process. Such documentation is required by Joint Commission Medication Management [MM] Standard MM.08.01.01, Element of Performance (EP) 1, and you will need those data to evaluate how well the process is working and implement necessary actions to improve the process. It's best to build regular reporting of medication management data into all components of the process in ways that make reporting and data collection easy. Collecting and organizing performance data are easier in the digital age, provided the information you

Collaboration

Data collection presents a great opportunity to collaborate with leadership and information technology professionals in your organization. There are a variety of digital health information systems available to organizations, such as electronic health record systems and digital ordering systems, some of which are highly customizable. Whether you work with an off-the-shelf solution or your organization has developed its own solutions, these systems are a primary source of performance data.

You can work with information technology professionals to see to it that your digital health information system allows for easy recording of adverse events. For example, you can use it to document how well storage and administration protocols are followed by staff. Many systems also offer options for recording patient monitoring activities and anything else you might want to analyze later. Get leadership involved to make sure that the resources are available to assist with the data collection you need to best analyze your performance.

want is regularly recorded in digital systems, such as electronic health records, pharmacy inventories and ordering systems, and supervisory reviews.

Quantitative vs. Qualitative Data

To get a full picture about what's going on inside your medication management system, you need to collect both quantitative and qualitative data. Quantitative data are objectively measured numerical data. Basically, quantitative data are the raw numbers that represent everything from medication error rates to the number of antibiotic prescriptions filled by the organization to patient census data. Anything that can be objectively quantified can become quantitative data. Analysis of quantitative data generally involves mathematical and statistical techniques to identify trends and other relationships and help make predictions.

Qualitative data are what can't be measured objectively but can lend context and insight to ideas and conclusions suggested by quantitative analysis. Examples of qualitative data include comments by staff during meetings or reviews, feedback from surveys or interviews conducted as part of a comprehensive review such as root cause analysis, clinical observations that are not readily quantifiable, and comments from patients. Qualitative data, although not objectively measurable, can be key to informing decisions suggested by the analysis of the numbers.

in other **words**

qualitative data

Data that are of, relating to, or involving the measurement of qualities, types, or kind; categorical information that cannot be counted, measured, or easily expressed using numbers.

quantitative data

Data that are of, relating to, or involving the measurement of quantity or amount; information expressed as numbers.

KEY CONCEPT

Analyzing Data

After you've made sure that you are collecting the data you need to get a picture of all the various parts of your medication management system, you need to analyze the data to identify patterns that can inform your performance improvement decisions. You might consider involving someone with a background in statistics or data analysis to help you make sense of what you're seeing. Data analysis can help you identify where variation is occurring and why and devise strategies to reduce or eliminate it.

Common Data Analysis Techniques

There are several data analysis techniques and tools available, and your organization likely has identified ones it prefers. Figure 8-4 on page 108 gives a description of some common tools. Note that there are plenty of examples and resources available online for these and other data analysis techniques.

in other **words**

data analysis

A process of inspecting, cleansing, transforming, and modeling data with the goal of discovering useful information, informing conclusions, and supporting decision making.

picture this

Figure 8-4. Data Analysis Tools

Regression Analysis	• A mathematical technique for identifying the relationship between two variables • **Example:** Used to find out what impact an increase or a decrease in antibiotic prescriptions has on rates of a health care-associated infection
Monte Carlo Simulation	• A technique for modeling the possible outcomes of a process and the probability of each • **Example:** Used to model the effects of drug interactions in patients
Factor Analysis	• The grouping of strongly correlated variables in a process to identify the links between them • **Example:** Used to identify and explore the links between correlated factors such as age and adherence to a medication regimen
Cohort Analysis	• The extraction of a subset of a larger data set based on a common variable • **Example:** Used to analyze medication management data just for pediatric patients, just for opioid medication prescription, or just for overnight shifts
Cluster Analysis	• The grouping of like data together and the separating of unlike data. Cluster analysis helps make sense of large data sets by breaking them down into groups of similar events or phenomena. • **Example:** Used to identify categories of patients who do or do not respond to a given medication or therapy, which could help explain why some do and some do not

These and other data analysis techniques can help you assess various aspects of your medication management system.

Comparing Data

Comparing data can help you identify risk points in your medication management process by establishing baseline performance levels, patterns, and trends. Data comparison is really another kind of data analysis.

Organizations compare data in many useful ways. For instance, you can compare performance data over time, which is a critical tool for assessing whether performance improvement initiatives are having the desired effect. Another option is to compare data from different times of the year, or throughout the day, to detect seasonal or other time-based variations and patterns. You can also compare data over longer periods to identify cyclical patterns. And you can compare your organization's data to other available similar data sets, such as state, regional, or national data from government sources or journal articles.

TRY THIS TOOL

Tool 8-2. Data Collection and Analysis Worksheet

Use this worksheet to identify the basics of data collection and analysis and establish measurements for your collection efforts.

in other words

risk point

A point in a process where the risk of variation is elevated.

KEY CONCEPT

Identifying and Addressing Improvement Opportunities

Now that you've collected and analyzed performance data related to your medication management processes, you're ready to put it to use. Every organization has room for improvement, and the constant striving for improvement is a hallmark of high reliability organizations. Take what you've learned from analyzing your performance data and use it to inform your decisions about what parts of your medication management system could use improvement and how you will go about trying to improve them.

Consider the following when thinking about performance improvement projects:

- **Patient safety.** Obviously, patient safety should be your primary concern. Prioritize improvements that analysis suggests will have the greatest positive impact on patient safety. Consider using a risk assessment matrix (see Tool 8-3 on page 111) to help you understand the scope and severity of different patient safety issues.
- **Sentinel event data and information.** If The Joint Commission has issued a *Sentinel Event Alert* (https://www.jointcommission.org/resources/patient-safety-topics/sentinel-event/sentinel-event-alert-newsletters/) on a topic related to medication management, that's a good place to start looking

to improve. The *Alert* itself should have helpful suggestions for improvement actions.

- **Other alerts and sources.** You can also identify areas of focus for your performance improvement activities by staying abreast of medication safety alerts issued by the Institute for Safe Medication Practices (ISMP), government agencies such as the US Food and Drug Administration (FDA), scholarly journals, and industry publications.
- **Setting-specific factors.** Each setting has its own set of compliance challenges, risk points, and areas of higher variation. These issues will be suggested by data and may also be identified in industry publications and scholarly literature.
- **Human factors.** Variation often can be reduced by designing systems or processes that make it easier for people to perform tasks in the desired way, such as creating digital order sets within your ordering system to ensure a greater degree of order accuracy and completeness.
- **Analysis of failures.** Use data and conclusions from a root cause analysis or another comprehensive analysis of adverse events.

in other words

high reliability organization

An organization that performs highly complex functions over extended periods of time without significant failures. These organizations typically prioritize safety over other performance measures. They are committed to resiliency and a high degree of situational awareness.

After you've identified areas of improvement, you'll want to work with leadership and others to prioritize improvement activities according to such criteria as the likelihood of patient harm, the simplicity or complexity of the intervention, alignment with the organization's mission, and others. Then you'll decide which improvement projects to pursue first. Take specific action to improve the process at the points given highest priority/highest risk in your analysis.

Smart Questions

What is your process for risk analysis?

How do you assess the likelihood and likely scope and impact of medication management process failures?

Implementing Performance Improvement Projects

There are many ways to go about implementing performance improvement projects, but most successful improvement projects tend to have a few things in common:

- Leadership buy-in
- Clearly defined goal and scope
- Use of performance improvement tools to examine a process, identify failure points, and redesign the process to address failure points
- Well-designed implementation plan
- Clear education plan for staff affected by changes
- Plan to monitor the system or process to see if changes are having the desired effects
- Plan to sustain positive effects over time

During periodic reviews of the medication management process, you should assess whether the projects you have implemented are producing the desired results by again comparing data over time. Note that engaging in performance improvement activities that overlap in area or scope may make it difficult to tell which activity is producing what effect. Be methodical in how you apply potential solutions. See if one thing works before trying another, or your data may be muddled.

When you have successfully implemented a positive change that addresses a specific area for improvement identified in your analysis phase, you can then think about ways in which the kind of fix you applied in this instance might be applied to other processes or systems in your medication management system or more broadly across the organization. This broader, second-order change requires more commitment on the part of leadership, but it can have far-reaching positive effects, including contributing to safety culture.

Performance improvement is a continuous process that has a goal of high reliability, which has no real end point (see Figure 8-5 on page 112). Understanding that performance and consistency can always be improved is foundational to safety culture. Encourage your staff to engage actively with this process by suggesting areas for improvement, helping to design improvement projects, and being proactive about reporting problems when they see them.

Continue to monitor performance to make sure improvement activities have the desired results and that the results are sustained. If not, you'll have further opportunities to improve. Again, analyze data to try to understand why the desired improvements didn't happen. Try another solution. Also, consider evaluating the review process itself to ensure that you are collecting the right quantitative or qualitative data, analyzing them effectively, and prioritizing the appropriate projects.

Smart Questions

What metrics do you use to assess how effective your performance improvement measures are?

TRY THIS TOOL

Tool 8-3. Risk Assessment Matrix

Use this risk assessment matrix to assess and prioritize risks in your organization's activities.

picture this

Figure 8-5. Performance Improvement as a Continuous Process

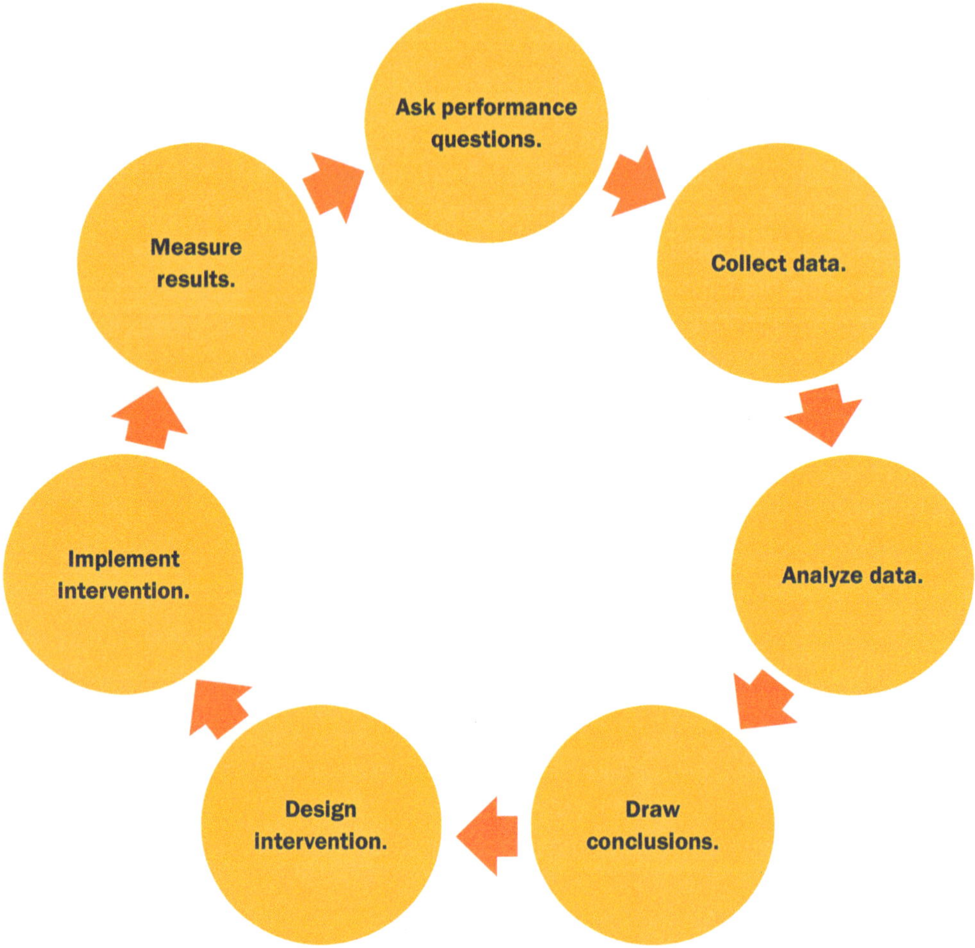

Ask performance questions.
Collect data.
Analyze data.
Draw conclusions.
Design intervention.
Implement intervention.
Measure results.

Follow these steps to keep the performance improvement process for medication management—and all areas of your organization—an ongoing process.

Additional Resources

- The US Food and Drug Administration (FDA) has a fillable PDF form used for the voluntary reporting of adverse drug events (https://www.fda.gov/media/76299/download). It also offers a webpage on the latest medication alerts and statements (https://www.fda.gov/drugs/drug-safety-and-availability/drug-alerts-and-statements).
- The Institute for Safe Medication Practices has *Medication Safety Alert!* newsletters that collect data from the error reports received through the National Medication Errors Reporting Program and National Vaccine Errors Reporting Program. https://www.ismp.org/newsletters
- The Joint Commission's Performance Improvement area offers tools and solutions to help with your organization's journey toward high reliability. https://www.jointcommission.org/performance-improvement/

CHAPTER 9

Establishing an Antimicrobial Stewardship Program

Antibiotics can be extremely beneficial to some patients. However, research from the Centers for Disease Control and Prevention (CDC) suggests that about 30% of antibiotics administered in acute care hospitals in the United States are unnecessary or suboptimal. Furthermore, antibiotics can cause serious adverse reactions in about one fifth of patients.*

Overuse or improper use of antibiotics also contributes to microbial resistance, as bacteria evolve to become immune or less susceptible to antibiotic medications. The CDC estimates that nearly 3 million antibiotic-resistant infections occur each year in the United States.

To help organizations optimize their use of antibiotics, the CDC produced guidelines that outline the core elements of antimicrobial stewardship programs. This initiative covers all departments involved in the prescribing and/or administering of antimicrobial medications that seek to optimize the use of antimicrobials. Joint Commission Medication Management (MM) Standard MM.09.01.01 sets requirements for antimicrobial stewardship programs in hospitals, critical access hospitals, and nursing care centers (for ambulatory health care organizations, antimicrobial stewardship is addressed in Standard MM.09.01.03). The CDC also offers antimicrobial stewardship guidance for other settings.

KEY CONCEPTS

- Leadership's Commitment to Antimicrobial Stewardship
- Staff Education
- Antimicrobial Stewardship Program Elements
- Collecting and Analyzing Program Data

* Centers for Disease Control and Prevention. *Core Elements of Hospital Antimicrobial Stewardship Programs* 2019. Accessed Nov 19, 2021. https://www.cdc.gov/antibiotic-use/core-elements/hospital.html.

The Standards

Following are the relevant standards for the content in this chapter from your setting's *Comprehensive Accreditation Manual* or its E-dition® counterpart.

Standard	AHC	ALC	BHC	CAH	HAP	NCC	OBS	OME
MM.08.01.01 The [organization] evaluates the effectiveness of its medication management system.	X	X	X	X	X	X	X	X
MM.09.01.01 The [organization] has an antimicrobial stewardship program based on current scientific literature.	X*			X	X	X		

AHC, Ambulatory Health Care; ALC, Assisted Living Community; BHC, Behavioral Health Care and Human Services; CAH, Critical Access Hospital; HAP, Hospital; MM, Medication Management; NCC, Nursing Care Center; OBS, Office-Based Surgery Practice; OME, Home Care.

* Antimicrobial stewardship requirements are addressed in MM.09.01.03.

The health care and human services fields are vast and provide care, treatment, and services to many individuals who may be referred to as patients, individuals served, residents, consumers, or clients. The term patient *is used throughout this book to describe a recipient of care, treatment, and services.*

KEY CONCEPT

Leadership's Commitment to Antimicrobial Stewardship

As with many areas in health care, a solid antimicrobial stewardship program begins with leadership commitment. Your organization's leadership can take steps to help create, support, and nurture an antimicrobial stewardship program and ultimately show its commitment to creating a safe environment for medication use. For example, leaders might support the creation of antimicrobial use accountability documents that can help staff and managers understand their responsibilities, provide resources (and funding) to optimize antibiotic use, task information technology with creating useful reports, leverage support when there is resistance to change among staff, and so forth.

Although antimicrobial stewardship programs often pay for themselves by reducing costs directly and indirectly related to antibiotics, leaders can make explicit budgetary commitments to the program so that everyone knows they have the resources necessary to carry out the goals of the program. And because optimizing antibiotic use can be tied to infection prevention and control, leaders can support the antimicrobial stewardship program by reviewing and supporting improvements to infection prevention and control efforts.

With input from physicians, leaders can also support antimicrobial stewardship efforts by setting clear performance improvement targets, support monitoring by including antimicrobial stewardship data in the electronic health record, and integrate antimicrobial stewardship and related performance improvement activities into the organization's strategic plans.

Leading Across Disciplines

Successful antimicrobial stewardship involves collaboration across the organization, including in the following areas:

- Pharmacists and pharmacy staff
- Infection prevention and control
- Quality assessment and performance improvement
- Medical staff
- Nursing staff
- Information technology

The individual(s) leading your antimicrobial stewardship program is responsible for making sure staff and operations are working together to optimize the organization's use of antibiotics. The individual(s) is responsible for designing the program according to nationally recognized guidelines, ensuring the commitment of leaders and managers across a range of disciplines, overseeing the education of staff and patients about antimicrobial stewardship efforts and practices (including the creation, when needed, of educational modules or other materials), and communicating and collaborating with staff and practitioners on antibiotic use issues.

KEY CONCEPT

Staff Education

Staff education is a big component of any successful antimicrobial stewardship program. Your organization needs to educate all staff members and prescribers who order, dispense, and administer antibiotics or monitor patients who have received them about antimicrobial resistance and best practices for antimicrobial stewardship.

In addition to ensuring that staff members understand the key goals of your antimicrobial stewardship program and what is expected of them in terms of practices and documentation, education topics might include the following:

in other words

antimicrobial resistance
The ability of microorganisms to resist and survive treatment with antimicrobial medications.

antimicrobial stewardship
The effort to measure and improve practices surrounding the prescribing and use of antimicrobial medications, with the goal of optimizing their use and reducing antimicrobial resistance.

Smart Questions

How do you know if your organization is using antibiotics efficiently and effectively?

Which antibiotics would you target in your antimicrobial stewardship program and why?

What is your organization doing to monitor antimicrobial resistance?

- Antibiotic resistance threats
- Benefits of antibiotic stewardship
- Risks and benefits of antibiotics
- Epidemiology of inpatient/outpatient antibiotic use and opportunities for improvement
- Communication training for clinicians to improve inpatient/outpatient antibiotic prescribing and use
- Antibiotic stewardship considerations for the management of common inpatient/outpatient conditions
- Antibiotic stewardship in the outpatient setting, dentistry, emergency departments, hospitals, and nursing homes
- Antimicrobial resistance patterns in the community and within the organization

Smart Questions

How often do you offer staff continuing education about antimicrobial stewardship?

How do you assess antimicrobial stewardship compliance?

According to MM.09.01.01, EP 5,* your organization is required to deliver this education. You can determine how frequently to offer refresher courses or continuing education. The timing may depend on performance data or changes in operations, patient population, or other factors specific to your organization or setting.

KEY CONCEPT

Antimicrobial Stewardship Program Elements

Let's dig into the core elements of an antimicrobial stewardship program. These are reflected explicitly in Joint Commission Standard MM.09.01.01.*

- **Leadership commitment.** Leadership demonstrates commitment to the program by dedicating the necessary human, financial, and information technology resources to it. People involved in the program, whether they are on the team or executing the protocols, need time, tools, and tracking. Leadership can make sure they get the resources they need.
- **Accountability.** The program should have a leader or coleaders, perhaps a physician and/or pharmacist, who is responsible for directing activities and achieving goals under the program.

* This is not a requirement for assisted living communities, behavioral health care and human services organizations, home care organizations, or office-based surgery practices. For antimicrobial stewardship requirements for ambulatory health care centers, refer to MM.09.01.03.

- **Pharmacy expertise.** Pharmacy expertise, or medication expertise, is an indispensable part of antimicrobial stewardship. Appointing a single pharmacist leader whose focus within the program is to keep working to improve antibiotic use in the organization can help make sure the program stays grounded in current science.
- **Action.** Any effective program needs some way of making sure its decisions and recommendations are acted upon.
- **Tracking.** Information about infection rates, antibiotic prescribing, antimicrobial resistance patterns, and other data relevant to the program informs the decisions and recommendations of the team. Organization and antimicrobial stewardship program leadership can work together to design a system of capturing the data they need and comparing data over time.
- **Reporting.** After your antimicrobial stewardship team has collected and analyzed program data, they may reach conclusions about trends in prescribing and antimicrobial resistance patterns. They can then communicate those conclusions to physicians, nurses, and other staff so they know how the program is working, what difficulties to look for, and the ways their own actions can contribute to the success of the program.
- **Education.** To instill the importance of working together, you've got to educate practitioners, nurses, and other staff on the value of antimicrobial stewardship and how they can advance the program's goals.

Be sure to familiarize yourself even further with the central concepts of antimicrobial stewardship (see Additional Resources on page 124). Start with the CDC's guidance on antimicrobial stewardship programs, and work to stay current with the literature about best practices in infection prevention and control and antibiotic use.

picture this

Figure 9-1. Core Elements of Antimicrobial Stewardship Programs

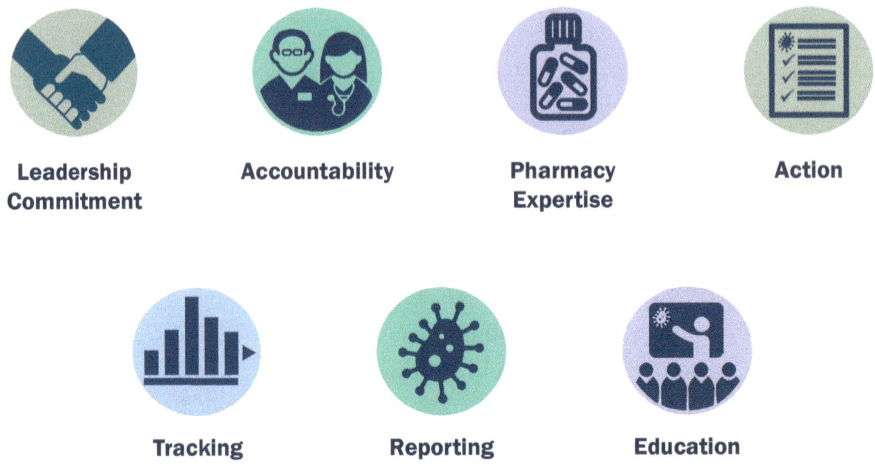

Source: Adapted from the Centers for Disease Control and Prevention. *The Core Elements of Hospital Antibiotic Stewardship Programs:* 2019. 2019. Accessed Nov 19, 2021. https://www.cdc.gov/antibiotic-use/healthcare/pdfs/hospital-core-elements-H.pdf.

TRY THIS TOOL

Tool 9-1. Antimicrobial Stewardship Program Checklist

Use this checklist to assess whether your organization meets the basic requirements for an effective antimicrobial stewardship program.

Multidisciplinary Team

An organization looking to set up or improve its antimicrobial stewardship program needs a multidisciplinary team to oversee the program (see Figure 9-2 on page 121). When possible, this team should include an infectious disease physician, one or more infection preventionists, one or more pharmacists, and one or more practitioners. If necessary, team members may be drawn from part-time staff, consultant staff, or telehealth staff. And it goes without saying that the team will need the participation and support of leadership to make sure that resources and time are made available to the team and its members.

picture this

Figure 9-2. Antimicrobial Stewardship Team

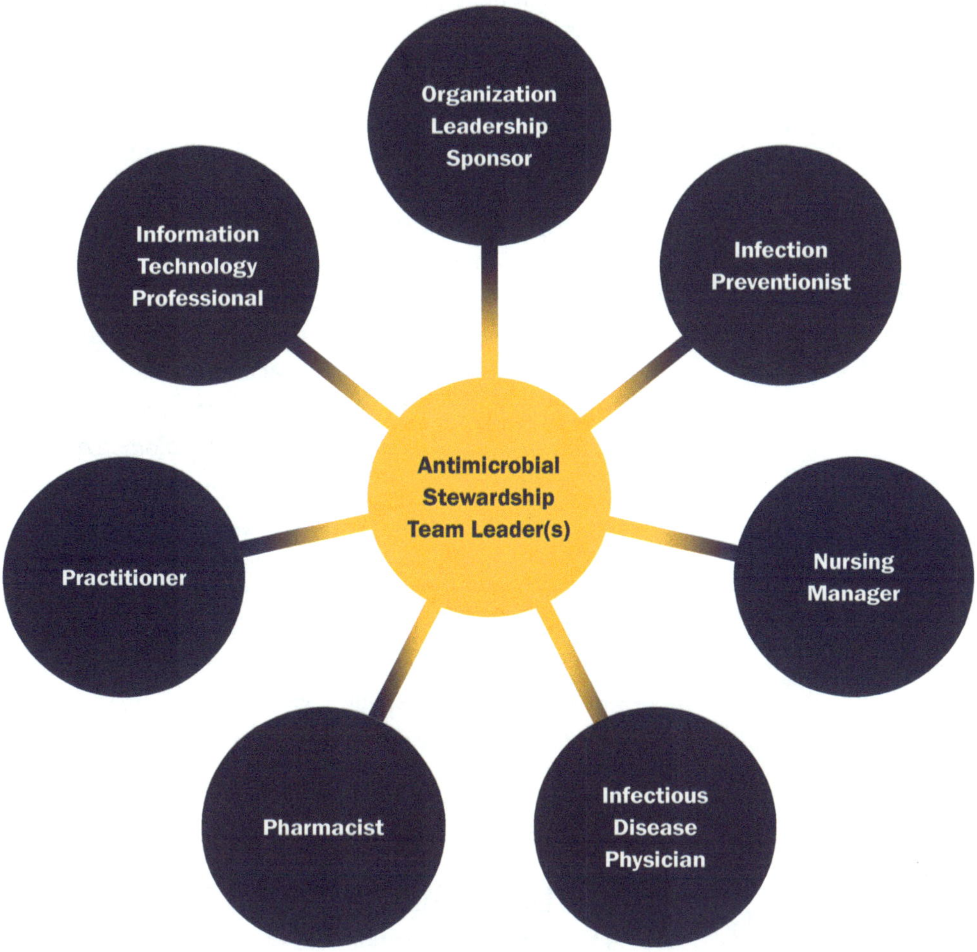

Organization Leadership Sponsor
Infection Preventionist
Nursing Manager
Infectious Disease Physician
Pharmacist
Practitioner
Information Technology Professional
Antimicrobial Stewardship Team Leader(s)

Antimicrobial stewardship is an organizationwide effort that touches every department involved in the prescribing and administering of antimicrobial medications. Therefore, an effective antimicrobial stewardship program requires the participation of a broad interdisciplinary team, including department leaders from across the organization.

in other words

infection preventionist

A health care professional whose focus is the prevention of infections associated with health care.

TRY THIS TOOL

Tool 9-2. Antimicrobial Stewardship Practice Checklist

Use this checklist to examine the practical application of the core elements of your antimicrobial stewardship program.

Smart Questions

What are the goals of your antimicrobial stewardship program?

What is the organization doing well?

Where is there room for improvement?

What data are you collecting that support your assessment?

Targeted Interventions

The goals of an antimicrobial stewardship program are to promote judicious use of antibiotics across the organization, to think critically about when antibiotics are the appropriate treatment, and to improve patient outcomes when infections do occur (see Figure 9-1 on page 120 for a list of core elements). Accomplishing these goals requires the work of your multidisciplinary team. Initially this work will take the form of developing multidisciplinary protocols. These include organization interventions, policies, and procedures that address the activities of staff and practitioners and that clarify their responsibilities under the program.

Examples of the kinds of interventions, policies, and procedures the team might develop or use include the following:

- Antibiotic formulary restrictions
- Assessments of appropriateness of antibiotics for a variety of infections, such as community-acquired pneumonia, skin and soft tissue infections, and urinary tract infections
- Protocols for care of patients with *Clostridioides difficile (C. diff)*
- Guidelines for antimicrobial use in adults and children
- Plan for parenteral to oral antibiotic conversion
- Preauthorization requirements for specific antimicrobials
- Guidelines for the use of prophylactic antibiotics

A multidisciplinary team that is familiar with the literature and current best practices will be able to decide which protocols they need to reach the program's goals.

KEY CONCEPT

Collecting and Analyzing Program Data

Collecting and analyzing data are critical to the success of any antimicrobial stewardship effort. Frontline workers and others involved in patient care need a system that allows them to easily report or record data on prescribing patterns, antimicrobial resistance patterns, infection rates, and other relevant measures. You then need a way to extract this data from recordkeeping systems already in use. The data collected and analyzed in this phase of the program are foundational to an evidence-based understanding and practice of antibiotic prescription and use. *See* Figure 9-3 on page 123 for an example of the process.

Examples of data to be collected include but are not limited to the following:

picture this

Figure 9-3. Sample Antimicrobial Stewardship Program Process

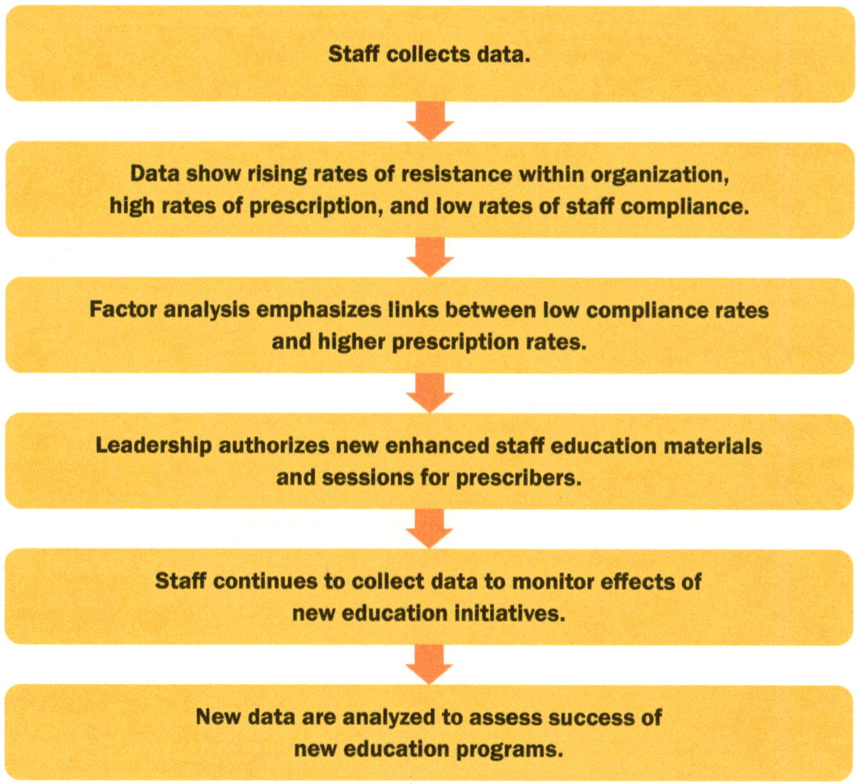
Staff collects data.
Data show rising rates of resistance within organization, high rates of prescription, and low rates of staff compliance.
Factor analysis emphasizes links between low compliance rates and higher prescription rates.
Leadership authorizes new enhanced staff education materials and sessions for prescribers.
Staff continues to collect data to monitor effects of new education initiatives.
New data are analyzed to assess success of new education programs.

This diagram shows an example of how the antimicrobial stewardship program might work to identify and address suboptimal antimicrobial prescribing.

- Antimicrobial prescribing rates and patterns
- Antimicrobial resistance rates and patterns
- Measures of staff compliance with the program
- Financial data related to antimicrobial medications and infection prevention and control interventions
- Measures of the delivery of staff education
- Measures of the delivery of patient education
- Changes in any measured program values over time

Smart Questions

Where are the data you need to track antimicrobial stewardship performance?

TRY THIS TOOL

Tool 9-3. Antimicrobial Stewardship Procedures

Use this sample set of procedures to inform your thinking about the procedures for your own antimicrobial stewardship program. Be sure to customize them to suit the needs and requirements of your organization.

You need to identify which data will tell you meaningful things about the program, collect and analyze them over time, compare the data to previous performance and evidence-based benchmarks from literature and government data sets, and set a course for improvement. And you need to monitor your improvement efforts to make sure your interventions are working and that their effects are sustained. These processes apply just as much to the antimicrobial stewardship program as to the broader medication management system.

There are several factors that go into developing and maintaining a successful antimicrobial stewardship program. With leadership commitment, staff education, and continuous monitoring and data collection, your organization has a better chance to optimize its use of antibiotics.

Additional Resources

- The Centers for Disease Control and Prevention (CDC) has a webpage on the core elements of hospital antibiotic stewardship programs (https://www.cdc.gov/antibiotic-use/core-elements/hospital.html). The CDC's National Healthcare Safety Network has a webpage dedicated to antimicrobial use and resistance options (https://www.cdc.gov/nhsn/psc/aur/index.html).
- The Association for Professionals in Infection Control and Epidemiology includes a number of resources on its antimicrobial stewardship webpage. https://apic.org/professional-practice/practice-resources/antimicrobial-stewardship/
- Johns Hopkins Medicine has created a Toolkit to Enhance Nursing and Antibiotic Stewardship Partnership. https://www.hopkinsmedicine.org/antimicrobial-stewardship/nursing-toolkit/index.html
- The Agency for Healthcare Research and Quality offers a Nursing Home Antimicrobial Stewardship Guide on its website. https://www.ahrq.gov/nhguide/index.html
- The Joint Commission has a number of resources related to antimicrobial stewardship. https://www.jointcommission.org/resources/patient-safety-topics/infection-prevention-and-control/antimicrobial-stewardship/

Applicable Medication Management Standards

Following are the relevant Medication Management standards for the content in *Medication Management Made Easy* from your setting's *Comprehensive Accreditation Manual* or its E-dition® counterpart. Please note that these standards and elements of performance (EPs) are in effect at the time of publication of this book. Please check your manual or E-dition for the most up-to-date version.

	AHC	ALC	BHC	CAH	HAP	NCC	OBS	OME
MM.01.01.01. The [organization] plans its medication management processes.								
	X	X	X	X	X	X	X	X
EP 1. The [organization] follows a written policy that describes that the following information about the patient is accessible to licensed independent practitioners and staff who participate in the management of the patient's medications: • Age • Sex • Diagnoses • Allergies • Sensitivities • Current medications • Height and weight (when necessary) • Pregnancy and lactation information (when necessary) • Laboratory results (when necessary) • Any additional information required by the organization Note 1: This element of performance does not apply in emergency situations. Note 2: This element of performance is also applicable to sample medications.								

	AHC	ALC	BHC	CAH	HAP	NCC	OBS	OME
MM.01.01.03. The [organization] safely manages high-alert and hazardous medications.	X	X	X	X	X	X	X	X

EP 1. The [organization] identifies, in writing, its high-alert and hazardous medications.
Note: This element of performance is also applicable to sample medications.

EP 2. The [organization] follows a process for managing high-alert and hazardous medications.
Note: This element of performance is also applicable to sample medications.

EP 5. [For hospitals that use Joint Commission accreditation for deemed status purposes:] The [hospital] reports abuses and losses of controlled substances, in accordance with law and regulation, to the individual responsible for the pharmacy department or service and, as appropriate, to the chief executive.
Note: This element of performance is also applicable to sample medications.

	AHC	ALC	BHC	CAH	HAP	NCC	OBS	OME
MM.01.02.01. The [organization] addresses the safe use of look-alike/sound-alike medications.	X	X	X	X	X	X	X	X

EP 1. The [organization] develops a list of look-alike/sound-alike medications it stores, dispenses, or administers.
Note 1: One source of look-alike/sound-alike medication name pairs is the Institute for Safe Medication Practices (https://www.ismp.org/recommendations/confused-drug-names-list).
Note 2: This element of performance is also applicable to sample medications.

EP 2. The [organization] takes action to prevent errors involving the interchange of the medications on its list of look-alike/sound-alike medications.
Note: This element of performance is also applicable to sample medications.

EP 3. The [organization] annually reviews and, as necessary, revises its list of look-alike/sound-alike medications.
Note: This element of performance is also applicable to sample medications.

	AHC	ALC	BHC	CAH	HAP	NCC	OBS	OME
MM.02.01.01. The [organization] selects and procures medications.	X		X	X	X		X	X

EP 1. Members of the medical staff, licensed independent practitioners, pharmacists, and staff involved in ordering, dispensing, administering, and/or monitoring the effects of medications develop written criteria for determining which medications are available for dispensing or administering to patients.
Note: This element of performance is also applicable to sample medications.

EP 2. The [organization] develops and approves criteria for selecting medications, which, at a minimum, include the following:
- Indications for use
- Effectiveness
- Drug interactions
- Potential for errors and abuse
- Adverse drug events
- Sentinel event advisories
- Population(s) served (for example, pediatrics, geriatrics)
- Other risks
- Costs

Note: This element of performance is also applicable to sample medications.

	AHC	ALC	BHC	CAH	HAP	NCC	OBS	OME
EP 3. Before using a medication new to the [organization], the [organization] determines a method to monitor the response of the patient. Note: This element of performance is also applicable to sample medications.								
EP 4. The [organization] maintains a formulary, including medication strength and dosage. The formulary is readily available to those involved in medication management. Note 1: Sample medications are not required to be on the formulary. Note 2: In some settings, the term "list of medications available for use" is used instead of "formulary." The terms are synonymous.								
EP 6. The [organization] standardizes and limits the number of drug concentrations available to meet patient care needs.								
EP 7. The [organization] follows a process to select, approve, and procure medications that are not on its formulary. Note: This element of performance is also applicable to sample medications.								
EP 9. Medications designated as available for dispensing or administration are reviewed at least annually based on emerging safety and efficacy information.								
EP 10. The [organization] follows a process to communicate medication shortages and outages to licensed independent practitioners and staff who participate in medication management.								
EP 12. The [organization] follows written medication substitution protocols to be used in the event of a medication shortage or outage.								
EP 14. The [organization] follows a process to communicate the medication substitution protocols for shortages or outages to licensed independent practitioners and staff who participate in medication management.								
MM.03.01.01. The [organization] safely stores medications.								
	X	X	X	X	X	X	X	X
EP 2. The [organization] stores medications according to the manufacturers' recommendations or, in the absence of such recommendations, according to a pharmacist's instructions. Note: This element of performance is also applicable to sample medications.								
EP 3. The [organization] stores all medications and biologicals, including controlled (scheduled) medications, in a secured area to prevent diversion, and locked when necessary, in accordance with law and regulation. Note 1: Scheduled medications include those listed in Schedules II–V of the Comprehensive Drug Abuse Prevention and Control Act of 1970. Note 2: This element of performance is also applicable to sample medications.								
EP 4. The [organization] follows a written policy addressing the control of medication between receipt by an individual health care provider and administration of the medication, including safe storage, handling, wasting, security, disposition, and return to storage. Note: This element of performance is also applicable to sample medications.								
EP 6. The [organization] prevents unauthorized individuals from obtaining medications in accordance with its policy and law and regulation. Note: This element of performance is also applicable to sample medications.								

	AHC	ALC	BHC	CAH	HAP	NCC	OBS	OME
EP 7. All stored medications and the components used in their preparation are labeled with the contents, expiration date, and any applicable warnings. Note: This element of performance is also applicable to sample medications. **EP 8.** The [organization] removes all expired, damaged, and/or contaminated medications and stores them separately from medications available for administration. Note: This element of performance is also applicable to sample medications. **EP 9.** The [organization] keeps concentrated electrolytes present in patient care areas only when patient safety necessitates their immediate use, and precautions are used to prevent inadvertent administration. **EP 18.** The [organization] periodically inspects all medication storage areas. Note: This element of performance is also applicable to sample medications. **EP 19.** [For hospitals that use Joint Commission accreditation for deemed status purposes:] The [hospital] has a pharmacy directed by a registered pharmacist or a supervised drug storage area, in accordance with law and regulation. Note: This element of performance is also applicable to sample medications. **EP 24.** [For hospitals that use Joint Commission accreditation for deemed status purposes:] The [hospital] maintains records of the receipt and disposition of radiopharmaceuticals.								
MM.03.01.03. The [organization] safely manages emergency medications.								
	X	X	X	X	X	X	X	X
EP 1. [Organization] leaders, in conjunction with members of the medical staff and licensed independent practitioners, decide which emergency medications and their associated supplies will be readily accessible in patient care areas based on the population served. Whenever possible, emergency medications are available in unit-dose, age-specific, and ready-to-administer forms. **EP 6.** When emergency medications or supplies are used or expired, the [organization] replaces them as soon as possible to maintain a full stock.								
MM.03.01.05. The [organization] safely controls medications brought into the [organization] by patients, their families, or licensed independent practitioners.								
	X	X	X	X	X	X	X	X
EP 1. The [organization] defines when medications brought into the [organization] by patients, their families, or licensed independent practitioners can be administered. Note: This element of performance is also applicable to sample medications. **EP 2.** Before use or administration of a medication brought into the [organization] by a patient, their family, or a licensed independent practitioner, the [organization] identifies the medication and visually evaluates the medication's integrity. Note: This element of performance is also applicable to sample medications.								

	AHC	ALC	BHC	CAH	HAP	NCC	OBS	OME
MM.04.01.01. Medication orders are clear and accurate.								
	X	X	X	X	X	X	X	X

EP 1. The [organization] follows a written policy that identifies the specific types of medication orders that it deems acceptable for use.

Note: There are several different types of medication orders. Medication orders commonly used include the following:

- As needed (PRN) orders: Orders acted on based on the occurrence of a specific indication or symptom
- Standing orders: A prewritten medication order and specific instructions from the licensed independent practitioner to administer a medication to a person in clearly defined circumstances
- Automatic stop orders: Orders that include a date or time to discontinue a medication
- Titrating orders: Orders in which the dose is either progressively increased or decreased in response to the patient's status
- Taper orders: Orders in which the dose is decreased by a particular amount with each dosing interval
- Range orders: Orders in which the dose or dosing interval varies over a prescribed range, depending on the situation or patient's status
- Signed and held orders: New prewritten (held) medication orders and specific instructions from a licensed independent practitioner to administer medication(s) to a patient in clearly defined circumstances that become active upon the release of the orders on a specific date(s) and time(s)
- Orders for compounded drugs or drug mixtures not commercially available
- Orders for medication-related devices (for example, nebulizers, catheters)
- Orders for investigational medications
- Orders for herbal products
- Orders for medications at discharge or transfer

EP 2. The [organization] follows a written policy that defines the following:

- The minimum required elements of a complete medication order, which must include medication name, medication dose, medication route, and medication frequency
- When indication for use is required on a medication order
- The precautions for ordering medications with look-alike or sound-alike names
- Actions to take when medication orders are incomplete, illegible, or unclear
- For medication titration orders, required elements include the medication name, medication route, initial rate of infusion (dose/unit of time), incremental units to which the rate or dose can be increased or decreased, how often the rate or dose can be changed, the maximum rate or dose of infusion, and the objective clinical measure to be used to guide changes

Note: Examples of objective clinical measures to be used to guide titration changes include blood pressure, Richmond Agitation–Sedation Scale (RASS), and the Confusion Assessment Method (CAM).

EP 6. The [organization] minimizes the use of verbal and telephone medication orders.

EP 7. The [organization] reviews and updates preprinted order sheets, within time frames it identifies or sooner if necessary, based on current evidence and practice.

EP 8. The [organization] prohibits summary (blanket) orders to resume previous medications.

EP 9. A diagnosis, condition, or indication for use exists for each medication ordered.

Note: This information can be anywhere in the medical record and need not be on the order itself. For example, it might be part of the medical history.

	AHC	ALC	BHC	CAH	HAP	NCC	OBS	OME

EP 10. The [organization] defines, in writing, the circumstances for which weight-based dosing is required for pediatric populations.
Note: This element of performance is also applicable to sample medications.

EP 14. The [organization] requires an order from a doctor of medicine or osteopathy or, as permitted by law and regulation, a hospital-specific protocol(s) approved by a doctor of medicine or osteopathy to administer influenza and pneumococcal vaccines.

EP 15. [For hospitals that use Joint Commission accreditation for deemed status purposes:] Processes for the use of preprinted and electronic standing orders, order sets, and protocols for medication orders include the following:

- Review and approval of standing orders and protocols by the medical staff and the [hospital]'s nursing and pharmacy leadership
- Evaluation of established standing orders and protocols for consistency with nationally recognized and evidence-based guidelines
- Regular review of such standing orders and protocols by the medical staff and the [hospital]'s nursing and pharmacy leadership to determine the continuing usefulness and safety of the standing orders and protocols
- Dating, timing, and authenticating of standing orders and protocols by the ordering practitioner or another practitioner responsible for the patient's care in accordance with professional standards of practice; law and regulation; [hospital] policies; and medical staff bylaws, rules, and regulations.

EP 21. [For hospitals that elect The Joint Commission Primary Care Medical Home option:] The primary care medical home has an electronic prescribing process.

MM.05.01.01. [A pharmacist] reviews the appropriateness of all medication orders for medications to be dispensed in the [organization].

	AHC	ALC	BHC	CAH	HAP	NCC	OBS	OME
	X		X	X	X	X	X	X

EP 1. Before dispensing or removing medications from floor stock or from an automated storage and distribution device, [a pharmacist] reviews all medication orders or prescriptions unless a licensed independent practitioner controls the ordering, preparation, and administration of the medication or when a delay would harm the patient in an urgent situation (including sudden changes in a patient's clinical status), in accordance with law and regulation.
Note 1: The Joint Commission permits emergency departments to broadly apply two exceptions in regard to Standard MM.05.01.01, EP 1. These exceptions are intended to minimize treatment delays and patient backup. The first exception allows medications ordered by a licensed independent practitioner to be administered by staff who are permitted to do so by virtue of education, training, and organization policy (such as a registered nurse) and in accordance with law and regulation. A licensed independent practitioner is not required to remain at the bedside when the medication is administered. However, a licensed independent practitioner must be available to provide immediate intervention should a patient experience an adverse drug event. The second exception allows medications to be administered in urgent situations when a delay in doing so would harm the patient.
Note 2: A [hospital]'s radiology service (including [hospital]-associated ambulatory radiology) will be expected to define, through protocol or policy, the role of the licensed independent practitioner in the direct supervision of a patient during and after IV contrast media is administered including the licensed independent practitioner's timely intervention in the event of a patient emergency.

	AHC	ALC	BHC	CAH	HAP	NCC	OBS	OME
EP 2. When an on-site pharmacy is not open 24 hours a day, 7 days a week, the following occurs: • A health care professional determined to be qualified by the [hospital] reviews the medication order in the pharmacist's absence • A pharmacist conducts a retrospective review of all medication orders during this period as soon as a pharmacist is available or the pharmacy opens **EP 4.** All medication orders are reviewed for the following: • Patient allergies or potential sensitivities • Existing or potential interactions between the medication ordered and food and medications the patient is currently taking • The appropriateness of the medication, dose, frequency, and route of administration • Current or potential impact as indicated by laboratory values • Therapeutic duplication • Other contraindications **EP 11.** After the medication order has been reviewed, all concerns, issues, or questions are clarified with the individual prescriber before dispensing.								
MM.05.01.07. The [organization] safely prepares medications.								
	X	X	X	X	X	X	X	X
EP 1. A pharmacist, or pharmacy staff under the supervision of a pharmacist, compounds or admixes all compounded sterile preparations except in urgent situations in which a delay could harm the patient or when the product's stability is short. **EP 2.** Staff use clean or sterile techniques and maintain clean, uncluttered, and functionally separate areas for product preparation to avoid contamination of medications. **EP 3.** During preparation, staff visually inspect the medication for particulates, discoloration, or other loss of integrity. **EP 4.** The [organization] uses a laminar airflow hood or other ISO Class 5 environment in the pharmacy for preparing intravenous (IV) admixture or any sterile product that will not be used within 24 hours. **EP 5.** [For hospitals that use Joint Commission accreditation for deemed status purposes:] Medications are prepared and administered in accordance with the orders of a licensed independent practitioner or other practitioner responsible for the patient's care, and in accordance with [hospital] policies; medical staff bylaws, rules, and regulations; and law and regulation. **EP 6.** [For hospitals that use Joint Commission accreditation for deemed status purposes:] In-house preparation of radiopharmaceuticals is done by, or under the supervision of, an appropriately trained registered pharmacist or doctor of medicine or osteopathy.								

	AHC	ALC	BHC	CAH	HAP	NCC	OBS	OME
MM.05.01.09. Medications are labeled.								
	X	X	X	X	X	X	X	X

EP 1. Medication containers are labeled whenever medications are prepared but not immediately administered.
Note 1: An immediately administered medication is one that an authorized staff member prepares or obtains, takes directly to a patient, and administers to that patient without any break in the process.
Note 2: This element of performance is also applicable to sample medications.

EP 2. Information on medication labels is displayed in a standardized format, in accordance with law and regulation and standards of practice.
Note: This element of performance is also applicable to sample medications.

EP 3. All medications prepared in the [organization] are correctly labeled with the following:

- Medication name, strength, and amount (if not apparent from the container)
  Note: This is also applicable to sample medications.
- Expiration date when not used within 24 hours
- Expiration date and time when expiration occurs in less than 24 hours
- The date prepared and the diluent for all compounded intravenous admixtures and parenteral nutrition formulas

EP 7. When preparing individualized medications for multiple patients, the label also includes the following:

- The patient's name
- The location where the medication is to be delivered
- Directions for use and applicable accessory and cautionary instructions

EP 10. When an individualized medication(s) is prepared by someone other than the person administering the medication, the label includes the following:

- The patient's name
- The location where the medication is to be delivered
- Directions for use and applicable accessory and cautionary instructions

	AHC	ALC	BHC	CAH	HAP	NCC	OBS	OME
MM.05.01.11. The [organization] safely dispenses medications.								
	X		X	X	X		X	X

EP 1. The [organization] dispenses quantities of medications that are consistent with patient needs.
Note: This element of performance is also applicable to sample medications.

EP 2. The [organization] dispenses medications and maintains records in accordance with law and regulation, licensure, and professional standards of practice.
Note 1: Dispensing practices and recordkeeping include antidiversion strategies.
Note 2: This element of performance is also applicable to sample medications.

EP 3. The [organization] dispenses medications within time frames it defines to meet patient needs.

EP 4. Medications are dispensed in the most ready-to-administer forms commercially available and, if feasible, in unit doses that have been repackaged by the pharmacy or licensed repackager.

<table>
<tr><th></th><th>AHC</th><th>ALC</th><th>BHC</th><th>CAH</th><th>HAP</th><th>NCC</th><th>OBS</th><th>OME</th></tr>
<tr><td colspan="9">MM.05.01.13. The [organization] safely obtains medications when the pharmacy is closed.</td></tr>
<tr><td></td><td></td><td></td><td>X</td><td>X</td><td>X</td><td></td><td></td><td>X</td></tr>
<tr><td colspan="9">EP 1. The [organization] follows a process for providing medications to meet patient needs when the pharmacy is closed.

EP 2. When non-pharmacist health care professionals are allowed by law or regulation to obtain medications after the pharmacy is closed, the following occurs:
• Medications available are limited to those approved by the [organization].
• The [organization] stores and secures the medications approved for use outside of the pharmacy.
• Only trained, designated prescribers and nurses are permitted access to approved medications
• Quality control procedures (such as an independent second check by another individual or a secondary verification built into the system such as bar coding) are in place to prevent medication retrieval errors.
• The [organization] arranges for a qualified pharmacist to be available either on-call or at another location (for example, at another organization that has 24-hour pharmacy service) to answer questions or provide medications beyond those accessible to non-pharmacy staff.</td></tr>
<tr><td colspan="9">MM.05.01.17. The [organization] follows a process to retrieve recalled or discontinued medications.</td></tr>
<tr><td></td><td>X</td><td></td><td>X</td><td>X</td><td>X</td><td>X</td><td>X</td><td>X</td></tr>
<tr><td colspan="9">EP 1. The [organization] follows a written policy describing how it will retrieve and handle medications within the [organization] that are recalled or discontinued for safety reasons by the manufacturer or the US Food and Drug Administration (FDA).
Note: This element of performance is also applicable to sample medications.

EP 3. When a medication is recalled or discontinued for safety reasons by the manufacturer or the US Food and Drug Administration (FDA), the [organization] notifies the prescribers and those who dispense or administer the medication.
Note: This element of performance is also applicable to sample medications.

EP 4. When required by law and regulation or [organization] policy, the [organization] informs patients that their medication has been recalled or discontinued for safety reasons by the manufacturer or the US Food and Drug Administration (FDA).
Note: This element of performance is also applicable to sample medications.</td></tr>
<tr><td colspan="9">MM.05.01.19. The [organization] safely manages returned medications.</td></tr>
<tr><td></td><td>X</td><td>X</td><td>X</td><td>X</td><td>X</td><td>X</td><td></td><td>X</td></tr>
<tr><td colspan="9">EP 1. The [organization] determines under what circumstances unused, expired, or returned medications will be managed by the pharmacy or the [organization].
Note: This element of performance is also applicable to sample medications.

EP 2. When the [organization] accepts unused, expired, or returned medications, it follows a process for returning medications to the pharmacy's control which includes procedures for preventing diversion.
Note: This element of performance is also applicable to sample medications.

EP 3. The [organization] determines if and when outside sources are used for destruction of medications.
Note: This element of performance is also applicable to sample medications.</td></tr>
</table>

<table>
<tr><th></th><th>AHC</th><th>ALC</th><th>BHC</th><th>CAH</th><th>HAP</th><th>NCC</th><th>OBS</th><th>OME</th></tr>
<tr><td colspan="9">MM.06.01.01. The [organization] safely administers medications.</td></tr>
<tr><td></td><td>X</td><td>X</td><td>X</td><td>X</td><td>X</td><td>X</td><td>X</td><td>X</td></tr>
<tr><td colspan="9">EP 1. Only authorized licensed independent practitioners and clinical staff administer medications. The [organization] defines, in writing, those who are authorized to administer medication, with or without supervision, in accordance with law and regulation.
Note: This does not prohibit self-administration of medications by patients, when indicated.

EP 3. Before administration, the individual administering the medication does the following:
• Verifies that the medication selected matches the medication order and product label
• Visually inspects the medication for particulates, discoloration, or other loss of integrity
• Verifies that the medication has not expired
• Verifies that no contraindications exist
• Verifies that the medication is being administered at the proper time, in the prescribed dose, and by the correct route
• Discusses any unresolved concerns about the medication with the patient's licensed independent practitioner, prescriber (if different from the licensed independent practitioner), and/or staff involved with the patient's care, treatment, and services

EP 9. Before administering a new medication, the patient or family is informed about any potential clinically significant adverse drug reactions or other concerns regarding administration of a new medication.

EP 13. Before administering a radioactive pharmaceutical for diagnostic purposes, staff verify that the dose to be administered is within 20% of the prescribed dose, or, if the dose is prescribed as a range, staff verify that the dose to be administered is within the prescribed range.</td></tr>
<tr><td colspan="9">MM.06.01.03. Self-administered medications are administered safely and accurately. Note: The term "self-administered medication(s)" may refer to medications administered by a family member.</td></tr>
<tr><td></td><td></td><td>X</td><td>X</td><td>X</td><td>X</td><td>X</td><td></td><td>X</td></tr>
<tr><td colspan="9">EP 1. If self-administration of medications is allowed, the [organization] follows written processes that guide the safe and accurate self-administration of medications or the administration of medications by a family member (refer to the Glossary for the definition of family). The processes address training, supervision, and documentation.

EP 3. The [organization] educates patients and families involved in self-administration about the following:
• Medication name, type, and reason for use
• How to administer medication, including process, time, frequency, route, and dose
• Anticipated actions and potential side effects of the medication administered
• Monitoring the effects of the medication

EP 7. The [organization] determines that the patient or the family member who administers the medication is competent at medication administration before allowing them to administer medications.</td></tr>
</table>

<table>
<tr><th></th><th>AHC</th><th>ALC</th><th>BHC</th><th>CAH</th><th>HAP</th><th>NCC</th><th>OBS</th><th>OME</th></tr>
<tr><td colspan="9">MM.06.01.05. The [organization] safely manages investigational medications.</td></tr>
<tr><td></td><td>X</td><td></td><td>X</td><td>X</td><td>X</td><td>X</td><td>X</td><td>X</td></tr>
<tr><td colspan="9">EP 1. The [organization] follows a written process addressing the use of investigational medications that includes review, approval, supervision, and monitoring.

EP 2. The [organization]'s written process for the use of investigational medications specifies that the pharmacy controls the storage, dispensing, labeling, and distribution of investigational medications.

EP 3. The written process for the use of investigational medications specifies that when a patient is involved in an investigational protocol that is independent of the [organization], the [organization] evaluates and, if no contraindication exists, accommodates the patient's continued participation in the protocol.</td></tr>
<tr><td colspan="9">MM.07.01.01. The [organization] monitors patients to determine the effects of their medications.</td></tr>
<tr><td></td><td>X</td><td></td><td>X</td><td>X</td><td></td><td>X</td><td>X</td><td>X</td></tr>
<tr><td colspan="9">EP 1. The [organization] monitors the patient's perception of the side effects and the effectiveness of the patient's medication. Note: This element of performance is also applicable to sample medications.

EP 2. The [organization] monitors the patient's response to their medication(s) by taking into account clinical information from the medical record, relevant lab values, clinical response, and medication profile.
Note 1: Monitoring the patient's response to medications is an important assessment activity for nurses, physicians, and pharmacists. In particular, monitoring the patient's response to the first dose of a new medication is essential to the safety of the patient because any adverse reactions, including serious ones, are more unpredictable if the medication has never been used before with the patient.
Note 2: This element of performance is also applicable to sample medications.</td></tr>
<tr><td colspan="9">MM.07.01.03. The [organization] responds to actual or potential adverse drug events, significant adverse drug reactions, and medication errors.</td></tr>
<tr><td></td><td>X</td><td>X</td><td>X</td><td>X</td><td>X</td><td>X</td><td></td><td>X</td></tr>
<tr><td colspan="9">EP 1. The [organization] follows a written process to respond to actual or potential adverse drug events, significant adverse drug reactions, and medication errors.
Note: This element of performance is also applicable to sample medications.

EP 2. The [organization] follows a written process addressing prescriber notification in the event of an adverse drug event, significant adverse drug reaction, or medication error.
Note: This element of performance is also applicable to sample medications.

EP 3. The [organization] complies with internal and external reporting requirements for actual or potential adverse drug events, significant adverse drug reactions, and medication errors.
Note: This element of performance is also applicable to sample medications.</td></tr>
<tr><td colspan="9">EP 6. [For hospitals that use Joint Commission accreditation for deemed status purposes:] Medication administration errors, adverse drug reactions, and medication incompatibilities as defined by the [hospital] are immediately reported to the attending physician or clinical psychologist and as appropriate to the organizationwide quality assessment and performance improvement program.
Note: The definition of "physician" is the same as that used by the Centers for Medicare & Medicaid Services (CMS).</td></tr>
</table>

<table>
<tr><th></th><th>AHC</th><th>ALC</th><th>BHC</th><th>CAH</th><th>HAP</th><th>NCC</th><th>OBS</th><th>OME</th></tr>
<tr><td colspan="9">MM.08.01.01. The [organization] evaluates the effectiveness of its medication management system.
Note: This evaluation includes reconciling medication information.</td></tr>
<tr><td></td><td>X</td><td>X</td><td>X</td><td>X</td><td>X</td><td>X</td><td>X</td><td>X</td></tr>
<tr><td colspan="9">EP 1. As part of its evaluation of the effectiveness of medication management, the [organization] does the following:
• Collects data on the performance of its medication management system
• Analyzes data on its medication management system
• Compares data over time to identify risk points, levels of performance, patterns, trends, and variations of its medication management system
Note: This element of performance is also applicable to sample medications.

EP 5. Based on analysis of its data, as well as review of the literature for new technologies and best practices, the [organization] identifies opportunities for improvement in its medication management system.

EP 6. When opportunities are identified for improvement of the medication management system, the [organization] does the following:
• Takes action on improvement opportunities identified as priorities for its medication management system
• Evaluates its actions to confirm that they resulted in improvements
Note: This element of performance is also applicable to sample medications.

EP 8. The [organization] takes additional action when planned improvements for its medication management processes are either not achieved or not sustained.

EP 16. When automatic dispensing cabinets (ADCs) are used, the [organization] has a policy that describes the types of medication overrides that will be reviewed for appropriateness and the frequency of the reviews. A 100% review of overrides is not required.</td></tr>
<tr><td colspan="9">MM.09.01.01. The [organization] has an antimicrobial stewardship program based on current scientific literature.</td></tr>
<tr><td></td><td></td><td></td><td></td><td>X</td><td>X</td><td>X</td><td></td><td></td></tr>
<tr><td colspan="9">EP 1. Leaders establish antimicrobial stewardship as an organizational priority.
Note: Examples of leadership commitment to an antimicrobial stewardship program are as follows:
• Accountability documents
• Budget plans
• Infection prevention plans
• Performance improvement plans
• Strategic plans
• Using the electronic health record to collect antimicrobial stewardship data

EP 2. The [organization] educates staff and licensed independent practitioners involved in antimicrobial ordering, dispensing, administration, and monitoring about antimicrobial resistance and antimicrobial stewardship practices. Education occurs upon hire or granting of initial privileges and periodically thereafter, based on organizational need.</td></tr>
</table>

	AHC	ALC	BHC	CAH	HAP	NCC	OBS	OME

EP 4. The [organization] has an antimicrobial stewardship multidisciplinary team that includes the following members, when available in the setting:

- Infectious disease physician
- Infection preventionist(s)
- Pharmacist(s)
- Practitioner

Note 1: Part-time or consultant staff are acceptable as members of the antimicrobial stewardship multidisciplinary team.

Note 2: Telehealth staff are acceptable as members of the antimicrobial stewardship multidisciplinary team.

EP 5. The [organization]'s antimicrobial stewardship program includes the following core elements:

- Leadership commitment: Dedicating necessary human, financial, and information technology resources.
- Accountability: Appointing a single leader responsible for program outcomes. Experience with successful programs show that a physician leader is effective.
- Drug expertise: Appointing a single pharmacist leader responsible for working to improve antibiotic use.
- Action: Implementing recommended actions, such as systemic evaluation of ongoing treatment need, after a set period of initial treatment (for example, "antibiotic time out" after 48 hours).
- Tracking: Monitoring the antimicrobial stewardship program, which may include information on antibiotic prescribing and resistance patterns.
- Reporting: Regularly reporting information on the antimicrobial stewardship program, which may include information on antibiotic use and resistance, to doctors, nurses, and relevant staff.
- Education: Educating practitioners, staff, and patients on the antimicrobial program, which may include information about resistance and optimal prescribing.

Note: These core elements were cited from the Centers for Disease Control and Prevention's Core Elements of Hospital Antibiotic Stewardship Programs (**https://www.cdc.gov/antibiotic-use/healthcare/pdfs/core-elements.pdf**). The Joint Commission recommends that organizations use this document when designing their antimicrobial stewardship program.

EP 6. The [organization]'s antimicrobial stewardship program uses organization-approved multidisciplinary protocols (for example, policies and procedures).

Note: Examples of protocols are as follows:

- Antibiotic Formulary Restrictions
- Assessment of Appropriateness of Antibiotics for Community-Acquired Pneumonia
- Assessment of Appropriateness of Antibiotics for Skin and Soft Tissue infections
- Assessment of Appropriateness of Antibiotics for Urinary Tract Infections
- Care of the Patient with Clostridium difficile (C. diff)
- Guidelines for Antimicrobial Use in Adults
- Guidelines for Antimicrobial Use in Pediatrics
- Plan for Parenteral to Oral Antibiotic Conversion
- Preauthorization Requirements for Specific Antimicrobials
- Use of Prophylactic Antibiotics

EP 7. The [organization] collects, analyzes, and reports data on its antimicrobial stewardship program.

Note 1: Examples of topics on which to collect and analyze data may include evaluation of the antimicrobial stewardship program, antimicrobial prescribing patterns, and antimicrobial resistance patterns.

Note 2: [For hospitals that use Joint Commission accreditation for deemed status purposes:] The antibiotic stewardship program documents the evidence-based use of antibiotics in all departments and services of the [hospital].

<table>
<tr><th></th><th>AHC</th><th>ALC</th><th>BHC</th><th>CAH</th><th>HAP</th><th>NCC</th><th>OBS</th><th>OME</th></tr>
<tr><td colspan="9"> EP 8. The [organization] takes action on improvement opportunities identified in its antimicrobial stewardship program.
EP 9. [For hospitals that use Joint Commission accreditation for deemed status purposes:] An individual(s) who is qualified through education, training, or experience in infectious diseases and/or antibiotic stewardship, is appointed by the governing body as the leader(s) of the antibiotic stewardship program. The appointment is based on recommendations of medical staff leadership and pharmacy leadership.
EP 10. [For hospitals that use Joint Commission accreditation for deemed status purposes:] The antibiotic stewardship program demonstrates coordination among all components of the [hospital] responsible for antibiotic use and resistance, including, but not limited to, the infection prevention and control program, the quality assessment and performance improvement program, the medical staff, nursing services, and pharmacy services.
EP 11. [For hospitals that use Joint Commission accreditation for deemed status purposes:] The leader of the antibiotic stewardship program is responsible for the following:
<ul>
<li>Developing and implementing a [hospital]wide antibiotic stewardship program, based on nationally recognized guidelines, to monitor and improve the use of antibiotics</li>
<li>Documenting antibiotic stewardship activities</li>
<li>Communicating and collaborating with the medical staff, nursing, and pharmacy leadership, as well as with the [hospital]'s infection prevention and control and quality assessment and performance improvement programs on antibiotic use issues</li>
<li>Training and educating staff, including medical staff, on the practical applications of antibiotic stewardship guidelines, policies, and procedures</li>
</ul></td></tr>
<tr><td colspan="9">MM.09.01.03. Antimicrobial stewardship is identified as an organizational priority.</td></tr>
<tr><td></td><td>X</td><td></td><td></td><td></td><td></td><td></td><td></td><td></td></tr>
<tr><td colspan="9"> EP 1. The organization identifies an individual(s) responsible for developing, implementing, and monitoring activities to promote appropriate antimicrobial medication prescribing practices.
EP 2. The organization sets at least one annual antimicrobial stewardship goal.
Note: Examples of antimicrobial stewardship goals may include decreasing the use of antibiotics to treat viral infections or addressing overuse of a specific medication.
EP 3. The organization uses evidence-based practice guidelines related to its annual antimicrobial stewardship goal(s).
Note: Guidelines may include diagnostic criteria and treatment recommendations to use when prescribing antimicrobial medications.
EP 4. The organization provides all clinical staff and licensed independent practitioners with educational resources related to its antimicrobial stewardship goal(s) and strategies that promote appropriate antimicrobial medication prescribing practices.
EP 5. The organization collects, analyzes, and reports data pertaining to the antimicrobial stewardship goal(s) to organizational leadership and prescribers.
Note: Data may include antimicrobial medication prescribing patterns, antimicrobial resistance patterns, or an evaluation of the antimicrobial stewardship activities implemented. </td></tr>
</table>

AHC, Ambulatory Health Care; ALC, Assisted Living Community; BHC, Behavioral Health Care and Human Services; CAH, Critical Access Hospital; HAP, Hospital; NCC, Nursing Care Center; OBS, Office-Based Surgery Practice; OME, Home Care.

Index

B

C

F

H

J

L

M

N

O

P

Q

R

S

T

U

V

W